Mastering Hypnosis

Alex Telman

Published by Alex Telman, 2024.

While every precaution has been taken in the preparation of this book, the publisher assumes no responsibility for errors or omissions, or for damages resulting from the use of the information contained herein.

MASTERING HYPNOSIS

First edition. December 8, 2024.

ISBN: 979-8227513489

Written by Alex Telman.

Table of Contents

Introduction

Welcome to "*Mastering Hypnosis: Complete Step-by-Step Manual, Case Studies, and Sample Scripts.*" Whether you're looking to explore hypnosis as a professional career or as a powerful tool for personal growth, this book offers you a comprehensive understanding of the craft and its transformative potential.

Hypnosis is often misunderstood, with many believing it's an arcane practice or something that only occurs in movies. In reality, hypnosis is a natural and effective way to access and work with the subconscious mind. It's a powerful tool for healing, growth, and achieving life-changing goals. By reading this manual, you'll not only learn the theory behind hypnosis but also discover practical techniques, real-world applications, and a detailed collection of sample scripts that you can immediately apply.

The **Manual** section of this book provides a step-by-step breakdown of hypnosis, from its historical roots to modern therapeutic applications. You'll learn how the mind works, how to induce and deepen hypnosis, and how to provide effective suggestions. Whether you are helping someone overcome stress, break a habit, or achieve greater confidence, this section will give you the foundational knowledge needed to practice hypnosis ethically and effectively.

The **Case Studies** section is an important part of this book, providing you with real-world examples of how hypnosis can be effectively applied in diverse situations. These case studies illustrate the transformative power of hypnosis in overcoming challenges, from breaking habits to overcoming deep-seated fears. By studying these examples, you will gain valuable insights into the practical application of the techniques you've learned, helping you refine your skills and deepen your understanding of hypnosis.

The **Sample Scripts** provide you with ready-made, tested scripts for some of the most common therapeutic areas hypnosis is used for. These scripts range from stress relief and relaxation to overcoming bad habits and boosting self-esteem. Each script is crafted to help you deepen your understanding of how hypnosis works and to provide you with practical tools to guide your subjects through a successful session.

Hypnosis is a profound journey, not just for the subject, but for you as the practitioner. It offers a unique way to connect with people on a deeper level, helping them to access their inner resources, heal past wounds, and achieve meaningful change. Throughout this book, you'll gain a deeper understanding of the power of the mind and how, with the right knowledge and skills, you can guide individuals to profound insights, relaxation, and transformation.

By combining the knowledge in the manual with the real-world case studies, and the hands-on experience of the sample scripts, this book equips you to master the art of hypnosis. Whether you are working with clients, friends, or even using hypnosis for personal self-improvement, this guide will serve as a valuable resource for many years to come.

As you move through this book, you will discover how hypnosis can help individuals break free from limitations, conquer their fears, and achieve goals they once thought impossible. It's time to harness the power of the mind, explore new possibilities, and use hypnosis as a force for positive change.

Let's begin this transformative journey together.

PART 1: GUIDEBOOK

Chapter 1: Introduction to Hypnosis

What is Hypnosis?

Hypnosis is a natural state of focused attention and heightened suggestibility, often accompanied by deep relaxation. It's commonly misunderstood, with many people associating it with magic, mind control, or a loss of control over one's actions. However, in reality, hypnosis is a therapeutic tool used to enhance a person's ability to concentrate and access the subconscious mind.

At its core, hypnosis is about entering a trance-like state, during which the individual is more open to suggestions, while still remaining in control of their actions. This state of focused awareness can be induced through various techniques, such as relaxation, guided imagery, or verbal suggestions.

What Hypnosis Is:

1. A Focused State of Attention
   When someone is hypnotized, their attention becomes sharply focused on a specific thought, image, or feeling. This concentration often leads to a diminished awareness of the surrounding environment, much like the intense focus you might experience when reading a book or watching a movie.
2. A State of Deep Relaxation
   During hypnosis, the body and mind often enter a deep state of relaxation. This can help reduce stress and anxiety, leading to an overall feeling of calmness.
3. A Tool for Behavioral Change
   Hypnosis can be used to help people overcome certain behaviors, such as smoking, overeating, or nail-biting, and can be applied to pain management, stress reduction, and even improving self-

confidence. It taps into the subconscious mind, where many of our habits and emotional responses are stored.

4. A Natural Mental State
    Hypnosis is not some magical, mystical experience—it is simply a natural mental state that people experience regularly. For example, you may have felt "hypnotized" while daydreaming, lost in thought, or deeply engaged in a task that requires intense focus.

What Hypnosis Isn't:

1. Not Mind Control
    One of the most common misconceptions about hypnosis is that it gives the hypnotist control over the subject's mind. This is false. The person being hypnotized cannot be forced to do anything against their will, beliefs, or values. A hypnotized individual is always in control and can refuse suggestions or exit the trance at any time.

2. Not Sleep
    Although the word "hypnosis" is derived from the Greek word for sleep ("hypnos"), it is not the same as being asleep. In fact, people under hypnosis are often very alert and aware, just in a deeply relaxed state. They can hear the hypnotist's voice and follow suggestions consciously.

3. Not a Magical or Mystical Experience
    Hypnosis is a scientifically understood process, and while it may feel like a "magical" experience to some, it's not about paranormal phenomena. Hypnosis works through psychological principles, and its effectiveness is rooted in the power of suggestion and the mind-body connection.

4. Not a Cure-All
    Hypnosis is a helpful tool, but it's not a magic fix for every problem. It works best when combined with other therapeutic methods and when used for specific issues like stress management, habit change, or emotional healing. It is not a cure for medical conditions, although it can be used as a complement to traditional medical treatments.

Hypnosis is a powerful tool that can help individuals access the subconscious mind, change habits, alleviate stress, and enhance overall well-being. It's a safe, natural, and scientifically recognized practice that allows people to tap into their inner resources to create positive change. Understanding what hypnosis truly is—without the myths or misconceptions—sets the stage for learning how to use it effectively. In the following chapters, we will explore the techniques and principles that make hypnosis a valuable skill for both personal and professional use.

Common Myths and Misconceptions About Hypnosis
Hypnosis has long been surrounded by myths and misconceptions, many of which are perpetuated by movies, TV shows, and popular culture. These misunderstandings often cause people to fear or dismiss hypnosis as something unnatural or even dangerous. In this section, we'll clear up some of the most common myths about hypnosis to help you better understand what it truly is.

Myth 1: Hypnosis is Mind Control

Fact: Hypnosis is not about controlling someone's mind or making them do things against their will. This is perhaps the most widespread misconception about hypnosis. While a hypnotist can offer suggestions to someone in a trance, the subject cannot be made to do anything that goes against their values, morals, or desires.

When you're hypnotized, you're in a highly focused state of attention, but you still retain control over your actions. You can choose to accept or reject any suggestion given. In fact, if a suggestion is uncomfortable or unethical, most people will not respond to it, even when in a deep trance.

Myth 2: You Can Be Hypnotized Against Your Will

Fact: You cannot be hypnotized unless you are willing to enter the hypnotic state. Hypnosis is a voluntary process, and people who are skeptical or resistant are much less likely to enter a deep trance. If you are unwilling or simply not open to the experience, you may not be able to enter hypnosis at all.

Hypnosis relies on the cooperation of the person being hypnotized. For example, someone who is actively resisting or doubting hypnosis may find it difficult to relax enough to achieve a hypnotic state. Therefore, consent and openness are key for the process to work effectively.

Myth 3: Hypnosis is the Same as Sleeping

Fact: While the word "hypnosis" comes from the Greek word for sleep, hypnosis is not the same as being asleep. In fact, a person under hypnosis is often more alert and focused than they would be in a normal waking state.

During hypnosis, the individual is in a relaxed yet highly focused state of awareness. They can hear everything happening around them and follow the hypnotist's suggestions consciously. This is why hypnosis can be used as a tool for therapy or behavior change—because the person is still actively engaged in the process.

Myth 4: People Can Reveal Secrets or Say Things They Don't Want to Under Hypnosis

Fact: While hypnosis can enhance a person's openness and suggestibility, it does not make someone reveal information they are unwilling to share. Hypnosis cannot force someone to disclose secrets or perform actions they are uncomfortable with. In fact, a person in hypnosis is still capable of resisting suggestions if they do not align with their values or wishes.

Hypnosis works with the subconscious mind, but the subconscious mind still follows the person's internal ethical guidelines. In other words, you cannot be made to reveal a deep secret or do something unethical while under hypnosis.

Myth 5: Only Weak-Minded People Can Be Hypnotized

Fact: This myth suggests that only people with weak wills or low intelligence can be hypnotized, but in reality, anyone who is open to the process can be hypnotized to some degree. Hypnosis is not a measure of strength or weakness—it's about the ability to focus and relax.

In fact, people who are intelligent, imaginative, and able to focus deeply are often more easily hypnotized because they can enter the relaxed, focused state more readily. Hypnosis has been shown to work for a wide range of people, regardless of their personality or intellectual capabilities.

Myth 6: Hypnosis is Dangerous and Can Cause Harm

Fact: Hypnosis is generally considered a safe and natural state when performed correctly. There is no risk of harm if the hypnosis is guided by a trained professional. While there are some rare instances of individuals experiencing mild side effects, such as dizziness or temporary confusion, hypnosis is not inherently dangerous.

It's important to note that hypnosis should always be practiced ethically by someone who is trained, especially in therapeutic settings. If done improperly or irresponsibly, any intervention could potentially have negative effects, but hypnosis itself—when done correctly—is no more dangerous than other therapeutic practices.

Myth 7: Hypnosis Can Solve All Problems

Fact: While hypnosis is a powerful tool, it is not a cure-all. Hypnosis can help with many things, such as stress reduction, habit change, and overcoming certain psychological blocks, but it is not always effective for every person or every problem.

It's important to have realistic expectations about what hypnosis can achieve. In some cases, hypnosis may need to be combined with other therapeutic practices for best results. For example, while hypnosis can help someone overcome a fear of flying, it might not be enough to address the root causes of that fear without additional psychological work.

Myth 8: You Will Do Something Embarrassing or Out of Control Under Hypnosis

Fact: Contrary to what is often shown in movies and media, people do not lose control of themselves during hypnosis. They are still in charge of their actions. The idea of a person clucking like a chicken or engaging in embarrassing behavior while under hypnosis is purely theatrical.

In reality, most people who are hypnotized simply experience a deep sense of relaxation, focus, and openness to positive suggestions. They may become more open to change or creative solutions to personal issues, but they will not lose control or engage in behaviors they wouldn't normally do.

Understanding the truth about hypnosis is the first step toward realizing its potential as a tool for personal development, therapy, and change. By clearing up common myths and misconceptions, we can see hypnosis for what it truly is—a natural, safe, and powerful state that can help people unlock their subconscious minds and create positive change in their lives.

History and Evolution of Hypnosis

Hypnosis, as both a concept and a practice, has a rich and varied history that spans thousands of years. Its development has been shaped by ancient beliefs, scientific discoveries, and evolving therapeutic practices. Below is a brief overview of how hypnosis has evolved over time.

Ancient Roots: Hypnosis in Early Civilizations

While the term "hypnosis" is relatively modern, the practice of using altered states of consciousness for healing or spiritual purposes dates back to ancient civilizations. Early forms of hypnosis-like techniques can be traced to the following:

1. *Ancient Egypt*
   The ancient Egyptians practiced rituals that involved inducing trance-like states to facilitate healing. They used sleep temples where priests would guide individuals into a deep state of relaxation, often combined with suggestion, to treat ailments.
2. *Ancient Greece and Rome*
   Figures like Hippocrates and Galen made early references to "magnetic" forces and the influence of the mind on the body. The Greeks also believed in divine healing powers, and some healing rituals likely involved hypnosis-like techniques, though not recognized as such at the time.
3. *India and China*
   Both Indian and Chinese traditions have long histories of practices involving meditation, concentration, and trance, often used for

healing, spiritual exploration, or relaxation. These practices share similarities with modern hypnosis, where focused attention and relaxation are key components.

The 18th Century: The Birth of Modern Hypnosis

The development of hypnosis as we know it today began to take shape in the 18th century. This era saw the blending of ancient practices with emerging scientific inquiry.

1. *Franz Anton Mesmer (1734–1815)*
   The father of modern hypnosis is often considered to be Franz Anton Mesmer, an Austrian physician who developed the theory of "animal magnetism" or "mesmerism." Mesmer believed that an invisible fluid, or magnetic force, flowed through the body, and that it could be influenced by a healer to restore balance and cure ailments. He would induce trance-like states by passing magnets over the body or through direct touch.

Although his theories were eventually discredited, Mesmer's work laid the groundwork for later developments in hypnosis. His practice of inducing a trance through suggestion and focused attention would evolve into what we now call hypnosis.

1. *The "Mesmerism" Movement*
   After Mesmer, many other practitioners adopted and expanded upon his ideas. However, the idea of "magnetic fluids" was controversial and eventually fell out of favor. Despite this, the practice of inducing trance-like states for therapeutic purposes continued to grow, particularly in France and England.

The 19th Century: Hypnosis as a Medical Tool

As the practice of mesmerism evolved, hypnosis became increasingly integrated into medical practice, especially in the treatment of pain and psychological conditions.

1. *James Braid (1795–1860)*
   In the early 19th century, the Scottish surgeon James Braid is often credited with coining the term "hypnosis" (from the Greek word "hypnos," meaning sleep). Braid rejected the idea of magnetic forces and instead believed that hypnosis was a state of focused attention, akin to concentration or intense relaxation. He also realized that it could be used to alleviate pain and treat psychological disorders, particularly in the context of surgery and anesthesia.

2. *The Rise of Hypnosis in Medicine*
   Braid's discoveries and contributions helped establish hypnosis as a legitimate tool in medical practice, particularly for pain management. During the 19th century, it became increasingly common for hypnosis to be used as an alternative to anesthesia in surgeries, especially during times when other anesthetic methods were not widely available or effective.

3. *Sigmund Freud and the Psychoanalytic Connection*
   Sigmund Freud, the founder of psychoanalysis, initially used hypnosis in his therapeutic work, particularly in the treatment of hysteria. He believed that hypnosis could be a useful tool for accessing repressed memories and emotions, a key component of his theories on the unconscious mind. However, Freud eventually abandoned hypnosis in favor of other therapeutic techniques, such as free association, although he acknowledged its potential for uncovering hidden psychological issues.

The 20th Century: The Scientific Exploration and Development of Hypnosis

By the 20th century, hypnosis had become more refined and scientifically understood, with growing interest in both its therapeutic and experimental uses.

1. *The Rise of Clinical Hypnosis*
   In the early 1900s, hypnosis began to be used more widely in clinical settings. Physicians, psychologists, and psychiatrists started

employing hypnosis to treat a variety of issues, including pain management, anxiety, and habit disorders. It was in this period that hypnosis began to be more commonly recognized as a legitimate therapeutic technique.

2. *Milton Erickson (1901–1980)*

   Milton Erickson, an American psychiatrist, is often credited with revolutionizing the use of hypnosis in therapy. Erickson's approach was marked by a deep understanding of the unconscious mind, and he developed techniques that focused on conversational hypnosis and indirect suggestion. Erickson's work made hypnosis more accessible to the broader public and showed its potential for treating a wide range of psychological issues, including phobias, anxiety, and depression.

3. *Scientific Studies and the Establishment of Hypnosis as a Psychological Tool*

   In the mid-20th century, the field of hypnosis began to see more rigorous scientific study. Research in the areas of neurobiology, psychology, and physiology started to provide a deeper understanding of how hypnosis works in the brain. The American Psychological Association (APA) recognized hypnosis as a valid psychological treatment in 1958, further cementing its role in both medicine and psychology.

The 21st Century: Hypnosis in Modern Practice

Today, hypnosis is widely used in various fields, including medicine, psychology, self-improvement, and even sports. It is no longer viewed as a mysterious or fringe practice, but rather as a scientifically supported technique for promoting mental and physical health.

1. *Hypnotherapy*

   Clinical hypnotherapy is a recognized therapeutic approach that integrates hypnosis with psychotherapy. Hypnotherapists are trained to use hypnosis to treat a variety of conditions, such as chronic pain, anxiety, stress, smoking cessation, and more. It is particularly effective in addressing deep-seated behavioral patterns and emotional issues.

2. *Hypnosis in Entertainment*
   Although hypnosis is widely recognized as a serious therapeutic tool, it also retains its place in the world of entertainment, often portrayed in stage shows where "volunteers" are hypnotized to perform amusing or extraordinary feats. These performances, while entertaining, are often based on highly suggestible volunteers and should not be confused with clinical hypnosis.
3. *Scientific and Neuropsychological Insights*
   Ongoing research continues to reveal new insights into how hypnosis affects the brain, particularly in relation to how it can reduce pain, manage stress, and alter cognitive processes. Neuroimaging studies have shown that certain brain regions are activated during hypnosis, particularly those involved in focused attention and sensory processing.

The history of hypnosis is one of gradual evolution, from ancient rituals to modern therapeutic practices. It has gone from being considered a mystical or magical practice to being scientifically validated as a valuable tool in both medical and psychological fields. Today, hypnosis is used for everything from pain management to behavior modification, and its acceptance continues to grow as more people experience its benefits firsthand.

Chapter 2: Understanding the Mind and Consciousness

Conscious vs. Subconscious Mind

To fully understand how hypnosis works, it's essential to have a clear understanding of the different levels of the mind: the conscious, subconscious, and unconscious minds. Each of these parts plays a significant role in how we think, behave, and experience the world around us. In this chapter, we'll explore the differences between the conscious and subconscious mind, as well as how they influence our thoughts, actions, and experiences.

The Conscious Mind

The conscious mind is the part of your mental processes that you are aware of in the present moment. It is the aspect of the mind that actively thinks, reasons, and processes information. It's where you make decisions, solve problems, and have direct control over your actions and thoughts. The conscious mind is essentially what you are experiencing right now—your active thoughts and awareness of your surroundings.

Key Characteristics of the Conscious Mind:

- *Awareness*: It is the seat of your awareness, meaning it processes information you are aware of in real-time.
- *Rational Thinking*: The conscious mind engages in logic, reason, and judgment, allowing you to analyze situations, make decisions, and solve problems.
- *Focus and Willpower*: The conscious mind is where you exert willpower and focus. You decide what you will pay attention to and what actions you will take.
- *Short-Term Memory*: It holds and processes information in short-

term memory. You can only actively hold and think about a limited amount of information at once.

For example, when you're reading a book or having a conversation, your conscious mind is actively engaged in interpreting words, understanding meaning, and deciding how to respond.

Limitations of the Conscious Mind: While powerful, the conscious mind can only handle a limited amount of information at once. It's often referred to as the "tip of the iceberg," as it only processes a small fraction of the total mental activity that occurs.

The Subconscious Mind

The subconscious mind, on the other hand, operates just beneath the surface of conscious awareness. It controls automatic processes, such as breathing, heartbeat, and other physiological functions. But it's not limited to just these functions—it also houses a vast reservoir of memories, beliefs, habits, and emotions that influence your behavior, often without you being consciously aware of them.

The subconscious is like a vast storage system, recording and holding onto information from your entire life, including experiences that you may not actively think about but that still affect your thoughts and actions. It also plays a key role in shaping your habitual responses and behaviors. In hypnosis, the goal is often to communicate with the subconscious mind to bring about positive changes, such as overcoming bad habits or emotional blockages.

Key Characteristics of the Subconscious Mind:

- *Automatic and Habitual Behavior:* The subconscious mind stores learned behaviors and automatic functions. It's what allows you to drive a car without thinking about every step or routine actions like brushing your teeth.
- *Emotional and Memory Storage:* The subconscious holds memories and emotional experiences, often shaping how you respond to current situations based on past events. For instance, a person who had a traumatic experience with dogs in childhood might feel nervous or

scared around dogs later in life, even without consciously recalling the event.

- *Influences Behavior:* The subconscious mind is responsible for many of your everyday actions, attitudes, and behaviors, particularly those driven by habit. It often operates in the background, influencing your thoughts and responses without your direct involvement.
- *Creative and Intuitive Insights:* The subconscious mind is also the source of your intuition and creative insights. Many creative breakthroughs and solutions to problems arise when you stop actively thinking about them and let your subconscious mind take over.

In hypnosis, the subconscious is often accessed directly to reprogram certain behaviors or beliefs. For example, someone might use hypnosis to alter a subconscious belief about their self-worth that's been holding them back in their personal life.

The Unconscious Mind

In addition to the conscious and subconscious, there is the unconscious mind. This aspect of the mind is considered the deepest level of mental processing, and it houses all of the thoughts, memories, desires, and experiences that are completely outside of conscious awareness.

The unconscious mind is thought to hold material that is repressed or buried, often because it's too traumatic, shameful, or otherwise difficult to confront. While the unconscious mind is not easily accessed, it can still influence thoughts and behaviors through deeper psychological mechanisms, such as dreams, slips of the tongue (called Freudian slips), and unresolved emotional issues.

In traditional psychoanalysis, therapists may try to bring unconscious material into the conscious mind in order to help a person process and heal from past trauma. However, much of the unconscious mind remains outside of our direct awareness and influence.

Key Characteristics of the Unconscious Mind:

- *Repressed Thoughts and Emotions*: It contains material that has been repressed—memories, experiences, and feelings that are too painful or uncomfortable to be processed by the conscious mind.

- *Instincts and Primitive Drives:* The unconscious mind also houses our basic instincts, such as survival instincts, sexual drives, and other primitive impulses.
- *Automatic Functions*: Much like the subconscious, the unconscious mind plays a role in controlling automatic functions, like regulating body temperature and digestion.

While hypnosis typically works with the conscious and subconscious levels, the unconscious mind can sometimes be accessed through deeper therapeutic techniques, such as psychoanalysis or advanced forms of hypnotherapy.

How Hypnosis Relates to the Mind's Different Levels

Hypnosis primarily works with the subconscious mind, helping individuals access deep-seated memories, emotions, and beliefs that may be affecting their thoughts and behaviors. Through relaxation and focused attention, hypnosis can help bypass the conscious mind and communicate directly with the subconscious, making it easier to reprogram unhealthy habits, thought patterns, or emotional responses.

For example, in hypnosis, a person may be guided to revisit a past event or trauma that they may have repressed or forgotten consciously, but which is still affecting them subconsciously. Once the subconscious mind is brought into awareness, the hypnotist can use suggestion to help the person release or change their emotional response to the event, thereby altering their behavior in the present.

Key Differences:

Conscious Mind:

- Active, aware, and focused thinking
- Controls decision-making and reasoning
- Short-tern, present-focused

Subconscious Mind:

- Stores memories, habits, emotions, and beliefs
- Influences automatic behavior, intuition, and creativity
- Long-term habitual, emotional responses

Unconscious Mind:

- Houses repressed memories and primal instincts
- Holds material that's out of awareness, often repressed
- Not directly accessible to conscious thought

Understanding the distinctions between the conscious, subconscious, and unconscious minds is essential for harnessing the power of hypnosis. By learning how the mind works at different levels, we can see how hypnosis can bypass the conscious mind and influence the subconscious to create lasting changes. The subconscious mind holds the key to many of our habits, beliefs, and emotional responses, and through focused attention, we can unlock its potential for healing, growth, and transformation.

How Hypnosis Affects the Mind

Hypnosis is a powerful psychological tool that directly interacts with the mind, particularly the subconscious, to influence thoughts, behaviors, and perceptions. It's not a mystical or magical phenomenon, but rather a state of heightened focus, suggestibility, and relaxation. In this section, we'll explore the mechanisms through which hypnosis affects the mind, including the physiological changes, brain activity, and psychological processes that occur during hypnosis.

1. Altered States of Consciousness

When a person is hypnotized, they enter an altered state of consciousness. This state differs from regular waking consciousness, as it involves a shift in attention, focus, and awareness. During hypnosis, the individual becomes deeply relaxed and focused on a specific thought, feeling, or sensation. Their peripheral awareness fades, and they become more receptive to suggestions.

Key Aspects of Altered States in Hypnosis:

- *Focused Attention:* The conscious mind becomes less active, and the individual's attention is narrowed to the subject at hand. This concentration helps filter out distractions, allowing deeper mental processes to take place.
- *Relaxation:* As the body relaxes, the mind also enters a state of calm, which can reduce stress and anxiety.
- *Increased Suggestibility:* The person becomes more open to suggestions, allowing the hypnotist to make positive changes in behavior, emotions, or perceptions. This heightened suggestibility is one of the core elements of hypnosis.

2. Changes in Brain Activity

Hypnosis has a measurable impact on the brain. Neuroimaging studies, such as functional magnetic resonance imaging (fMRI) and electroencephalogram (EEG), have shown that hypnosis can lead to changes in brain activity, particularly in areas involved with attention, relaxation, and mental processing. Some key findings include:

- *Increased Activity in the Anterior Cingulate Cortex:* This part of the brain is involved in attention, emotion, and decision-making. During hypnosis, this area often shows increased activity, which might explain the focused attention and heightened awareness that occurs during a trance.
- *Reduced Activity in the Default Mode Network (DMN):* The DMN is associated with self-reflection and mind-wandering. During hypnosis, activity in this network is typically reduced, suggesting that the individual becomes less focused on the self and more engaged with external suggestions.
- *Altered Sensory Processing:* Hypnosis can lead to changes in how sensory information is processed. For example, individuals may

report reduced pain perception, or they may experience sensory distortions (e.g., seeing an object in a different way or hearing a sound more clearly).

These changes in brain activity suggest that hypnosis creates a unique state of mind in which the brain processes information differently, enhancing the mind's ability to accept new suggestions and modify behaviors.

3. Dissociation: The Mind's Ability to Separate Awareness

One of the most interesting aspects of hypnosis is its ability to create a sense of dissociation, or the feeling that different parts of the mind can operate separately. This means that a person under hypnosis may experience a separation between their conscious awareness and certain mental functions or experiences.

For example:

- *Pain Dissociation:* In pain management hypnosis, a person may experience reduced pain sensation, even though their body is still in a state that would normally trigger pain. The conscious mind is able to disconnect from the sensory experience, making the pain less intense or completely absent.
- *Memory and Perception:* Hypnotized individuals may have altered perceptions of time, memory, or sensory input. For instance, they may forget certain details of an event or feel like time is moving faster or slower than usual.

This dissociative aspect of hypnosis helps individuals engage with their subconscious mind more directly. It allows them to access deeper memories or reframe emotional responses that are otherwise difficult to address while fully conscious.

4. Heightened Focus and Concentration

One of the most profound effects of hypnosis is the ability to significantly enhance focus and concentration. This is due to the deep relaxation and narrowing of attention that occurs during the hypnotic trance. People in this state can often focus on a specific suggestion or mental image with such intensity that their awareness of everything else fades away.

How This Affects the Mind:

- *Selective Attention:* Hypnosis allows individuals to focus on specific thoughts, sensations, or memories while blocking out irrelevant distractions. This can be especially helpful in therapies where clients need to focus on specific emotional experiences or negative beliefs.
- *Improved Mental Clarity:* Many people report experiencing mental clarity during hypnosis, as the relaxation and focus help reduce mental clutter and confusion. This enhanced mental state makes it easier to process emotions, confront fears, or work through challenging memories.

This intense concentration during hypnosis enables individuals to gain access to the subconscious mind, where deeply ingrained habits, beliefs, and emotions reside, allowing for more effective therapeutic intervention.

5. Reprogramming the Subconscious Mind

One of the primary goals of hypnosis is to influence the subconscious mind, where many of our automatic thoughts, behaviors, and emotional responses are stored. The subconscious is responsible for regulating habits, emotions, and long-held beliefs that shape our daily experiences.

During hypnosis, suggestions are delivered to the subconscious mind in a way that it can accept more readily. These suggestions can help change habits, beliefs, and emotional responses. For example:

- *Changing Habits:* Hypnosis can help individuals break free from bad habits, such as smoking or overeating, by implanting new positive suggestions into the subconscious mind.
- *Overcoming Fears:* Hypnosis can help reframe irrational fears or phobias by revisiting past traumatic experiences or creating new, positive associations with previously feared situations.

- *Increasing Self-Confidence:* Hypnotic suggestions can be used to build self-esteem and confidence by changing the negative beliefs stored in the subconscious mind.

By accessing and influencing the subconscious mind, hypnosis can make lasting changes to the way we think, feel, and behave.

6. Deep Relaxation and Stress Reduction

One of the most well-known effects of hypnosis is its ability to induce deep relaxation. This is achieved through a combination of focused attention, guided imagery, and physical relaxation techniques. This deep relaxation not only helps individuals feel calm and at ease but also brings about numerous benefits for mental and physical health.

How Relaxation Affects the Mind:

- *Reduced Anxiety:* The calming effect of hypnosis can help reduce anxiety and promote a sense of peace. This occurs because hypnosis reduces the activation of the body's stress response system, lowering levels of cortisol and other stress hormones.
- *Improved Emotional Regulation:* As relaxation takes over, people are better able to regulate their emotions. Hypnosis can help individuals process difficult emotions, such as grief or anger, by creating a sense of emotional detachment or reducing their intensity.
- *Better Sleep:* Many people find that hypnosis improves their quality of sleep by reducing stress and promoting relaxation. This is particularly useful for individuals struggling with insomnia or sleep disturbances.

Deep relaxation also aids in overall well-being by helping to balance the mind and body, making it easier to manage stress and navigate challenges more effectively.

Hypnosis interacts with the mind in a variety of ways, influencing mental states, brain activity, and subconscious processes. From altering attention and perception to reprogramming habitual behaviors and emotional responses, hypnosis works by creating a focused, relaxed state that allows for deeper access to the subconscious mind. By tapping into the mind's potential, hypnosis can be used to promote healing, facilitate behavior change, reduce stress, and enhance personal growth. Understanding how hypnosis affects the mind gives us insight into its incredible power as both a therapeutic tool and a tool for self-improvement.

Theories of Hypnosis

Hypnosis is a complex phenomenon that has been studied for centuries, and various psychological and physiological theories have been proposed to explain how it works. These theories attempt to understand the mechanisms behind hypnosis and why it can have such powerful effects on the mind and body. In this section, we will explore some of the most well-known and influential theories of hypnosis, including those that focus on dissociation, focused attention, and other psychological and physiological processes.

1. The Dissociation Theory

The Dissociation Theory of hypnosis is one of the most widely recognized theories. It suggests that hypnosis works by creating a state of dissociation—essentially a splitting or separation of different mental processes. According to this theory, hypnosis divides the mind into two parts: the conscious mind and the hidden, or "subconscious," part of the mind.

In a hypnotic state, the conscious mind is focused on the hypnotist's suggestions, while the subconscious mind becomes more open and suggestible. This dissociation enables the hypnotized person to separate themselves from certain thoughts, feelings, or experiences that might otherwise be overwhelming or difficult to process. For example, a person under hypnosis might experience pain relief or forget a traumatic memory temporarily.

Key Aspects of the Dissociation Theory:

- *Split in Consciousness:* The theory argues that hypnosis induces a split between the conscious mind (which is focused on the hypnotist's suggestions) and the unconscious or subconscious mind (which may store memories or emotions).
- *Altered Perception and Pain Control:* Under hypnosis, dissociation

can result in altered sensory perceptions, such as diminished pain or a sense of detachment from the body. For example, people undergoing hypnosis for pain management may report feeling that the pain is "numb" or "distant."

- *Memory and Emotional Detachment:* Dissociation also allows individuals to emotionally detach from stressful or painful memories. This is why hypnosis can sometimes be used for therapeutic purposes, such as overcoming trauma or phobias.

While the dissociation theory has been influential, some psychologists have critiqued it for oversimplifying the complex nature of hypnosis. However, it remains a popular explanation for certain hypnotic phenomena, such as pain management and memory retrieval.

2. The Social-Cognitive Theory

The Social-Cognitive Theory suggests that hypnosis is a product of social and cognitive factors, rather than a unique altered state of consciousness. This theory emphasizes the role of the individual's beliefs, expectations, and social context in determining the effects of hypnosis.

According to this theory, when a person is hypnotized, they are playing a role, similar to an actor in a play. The individual's willingness to comply with the hypnotist's suggestions and the expectations they have about the hypnotic experience significantly influence the results. In other words, hypnosis works because the person believes it will work.

Key Aspects of the Social-Cognitive Theory:

- *Expectations and Beliefs:* The theory suggests that people who believe in hypnosis are more likely to respond to it. Individuals with positive expectations about hypnosis may be more suggestible and, as a result, more likely to experience significant changes in perception or behavior.
- *Role-Playing:* In hypnosis, individuals may adopt a "role" in which they are expected to follow suggestions. This social role can help explain why some people are more susceptible to hypnosis than

others.

- *Social Influence:* The hypnotist's authority and the social context also play an important role in the effectiveness of hypnosis. The person being hypnotized may respond more strongly if they trust the hypnotist or if they are in a setting where hypnosis is expected to work.

This theory is supported by research showing that individuals with higher levels of fantasy proneness (the ability to imagine or daydream vividly) or susceptibility to suggestion tend to be more responsive to hypnosis. It aligns with the idea that hypnosis is more about the person's belief system and expectations than a distinct altered state.

3. The Focused Attention Theory

The Focused Attention Theory emphasizes that hypnosis is primarily a result of the individual's intense concentration and attention. This theory proposes that hypnosis is a heightened state of focus, in which the individual becomes highly absorbed in a single task or suggestion, with little attention to outside distractions.

When someone is hypnotized, their attention is narrowed to a particular experience or thought—such as a mental image or the voice of the hypnotist—and this intense focus leads to the hypnotic effects. This theory suggests that hypnosis is not an altered state of consciousness but rather an extension of ordinary mental processes like concentration and attention.

Key Aspects of the Focused Attention Theory:

- *Absorption in Task:* People under hypnosis are highly absorbed in the task at hand, such as focusing on the hypnotist's voice, following a visual suggestion, or imagining a scenario. This concentration results in reduced awareness of external stimuli.
- *Increased Suggestibility:* Because the person is so focused, they become more suggestible to the hypnotist's suggestions. This focused attention allows the person to experience changes in sensation, perception, and behavior, such as reduced pain or changes in

emotional state.

- *No Altered State:* This theory posits that hypnosis is simply an extreme form of focused attention, not a unique or altered state of consciousness. Instead of dissociation, it argues that hypnosis is an extension of normal mental concentration.

This theory is supported by research showing that individuals who are good at focusing their attention (e.g., people who are skilled at meditation or concentration exercises) are more likely to respond well to hypnosis.

4. The Neodissociation Theory

The Neodissociation Theory is a refinement of the Dissociation Theory, proposed by Ernest Hilgard in the 1970s. While the original Dissociation Theory suggests that hypnosis leads to a splitting of the mind into two distinct parts, the Neodissociation Theory proposes that hypnosis involves a complex interaction between different parts of the mind that works in concert, rather than a simple division.

According to this theory, hypnosis creates a state in which the individual's conscious awareness and the executive control functions (the parts of the brain that oversee behavior) are altered. Under hypnosis, these control functions become less dominant, allowing other parts of the mind, like sensory processes and memory, to operate differently.

Key Aspects of the Neodissociation Theory:

- *Altered Executive Control:* In hypnosis, the normal executive control of behavior becomes "dissociated" from awareness, meaning that an individual may carry out behaviors without conscious awareness or full control.

- *Hidden Observer:* Hilgard proposed that during hypnosis, there may be an inner "hidden observer" that monitors what's happening, even while the person may not consciously be aware of it. This explains phenomena like pain reduction or memory retrieval under hypnosis—where the conscious mind may not be aware of what's happening, but the subconscious mind is still processing the information.

- *Complex Brain Activity:* The Neodissociation Theory suggests that hypnosis works by creating a more flexible and dynamic interaction between different parts of the mind, rather than a simple split.

This theory accounts for the observation that some people may appear to be "unaware" during hypnosis (e.g., during pain management), yet still retain an underlying sense of observation or awareness.

5. The Physiological Theories of Hypnosis

Some theories of hypnosis focus on the physiological changes that occur in the body and brain when a person is hypnotized. These theories emphasize that hypnosis is a state that produces distinct physiological effects, such as changes in heart rate, muscle tension, and brain wave activity.

- *Relaxation Response:* One of the most prominent physiological theories is that hypnosis primarily works through the induction of a deep relaxation response, which helps reduce stress, lower blood pressure, and relieve muscle tension.
- *Brain Wave Patterns*: Research has shown that during hypnosis, individuals often exhibit brain wave patterns similar to those seen during deep relaxation or meditative states, such as theta waves (which are linked to deep states of relaxation and light sleep). This suggests that hypnosis can facilitate a deep state of relaxation, which may explain its therapeutic effects on conditions like anxiety and pain.

Physiological theories argue that these changes in the body and brain are what make hypnosis effective for therapeutic purposes, including stress reduction and pain management.

There are many different theories of hypnosis, each offering a unique perspective on how and why it works. From dissociation and focused attention to the influence of social factors and physiological changes, these theories help explain the diverse effects hypnosis can have on the mind and body. While no single theory fully captures the complexity of hypnosis, together, they provide a richer understanding of this powerful psychological phenomenon and its potential for healing and personal growth.

Chapter 3: The Hypnotic State

What Happens During Hypnosis?

Hypnosis is a unique and profound experience that affects both the mind and body in ways that are distinct from ordinary wakefulness or sleep. When a person enters the hypnotic state, a combination of physiological and mental changes takes place. These changes enable the person to become highly focused, relaxed, and receptive to suggestions, allowing hypnosis to be used for therapeutic purposes such as pain relief, behavioral change, and emotional healing.

In this section, we'll explore the physiological and mental transformations that occur during hypnosis, including the changes in brain activity, physical sensations, and cognitive processes.

1. Physiological Changes in the Body

While under hypnosis, the body experiences a deep state of relaxation that can result in several noticeable physiological changes. These changes can make hypnosis both a powerful tool for stress reduction and a therapeutic modality for managing pain, anxiety, and other conditions.

Key Physiological Changes Include:

- *Reduced Heart Rate and Blood Pressure:* One of the most significant physical effects of hypnosis is the reduction in heart rate and blood pressure. As the body relaxes, the parasympathetic nervous system is activated, which slows down the heart rate and dilates blood vessels, leading to lower blood pressure. This relaxation response is often used in therapeutic hypnosis to reduce stress and promote overall physical well-being.

- *Muscle Relaxation:* Muscle tension tends to decrease significantly during hypnosis. The body enters a state of deep relaxation where muscles loosen, which helps alleviate tension and discomfort. This effect is often harnessed in pain management, where a person can experience a reduction in pain or discomfort due to this muscle relaxation.

- *Changes in Breathing Patterns*: Breathing tends to become slower, deeper, and more regular during hypnosis. This change in breathing is a reflection of the relaxation and calmness that the individual is experiencing. The deep, slow breaths also help reduce stress by lowering the levels of stress hormones like cortisol.
- *Altered Sensory Perception:* Hypnosis can cause changes in sensory perception. For example, people may experience changes in how they perceive pain, sound, or visual stimuli. This is often used in therapeutic contexts, such as reducing pain perception or modifying unpleasant memories. Some people under hypnosis may even experience a temporary numbing sensation in a specific part of the body, which can aid in medical procedures.
- *Skin Temperature Changes*: A person in hypnosis may experience slight changes in skin temperature, particularly in the hands and feet. These changes are believed to be related to the relaxation of the blood vessels and a reduction in stress. Some hypnotists even use these changes to guide therapeutic interventions, such as enhancing relaxation further or inducing warmth to relieve pain.

2. Brain Activity During Hypnosis

Modern neuroimaging studies have provided valuable insight into how hypnosis affects the brain. Using technologies like functional magnetic resonance imaging (fMRI) and electroencephalogram (EEG), researchers have observed that hypnosis involves unique patterns of brain activity that distinguish it from ordinary wakefulness and sleep.

Key Changes in Brain Activity During Hypnosis:

- *Increased Activity in the Anterior Cingulate Cortex:* The anterior cingulate cortex (ACC) plays a key role in attention, decision-making, and emotional regulation. During hypnosis, the ACC becomes more active, which may explain the heightened concentration and focused attention that occurs during the hypnotic state. This increased activity can also contribute to the ability to ignore distractions and focus intensely on the hypnotist's suggestions.

- *Decreased Activity in the Default Mode Network (DMN):* The Default Mode Network is a collection of brain regions that are active when the mind is at rest or engaged in self-referential thoughts (such as daydreaming or reflecting on past experiences). During hypnosis, the DMN shows a reduction in activity, which may contribute to the sense of detachment from one's usual sense of self. This reduction in DMN activity helps explain why individuals under hypnosis can focus on suggestions and sensory experiences without being distracted by their normal internal thought processes.

- *Increased Connectivity Between Brain Regions:* One of the most notable findings in hypnosis research is the increase in communication between different regions of the brain. For example, there is increased communication between areas associated with sensory perception and areas that process emotions. This enhanced connectivity may explain the ability to change emotional responses or alter sensory perceptions (such as pain) during hypnosis.

- *Brain Wave Changes*: Hypnosis is also associated with changes in brain wave patterns. Typically, during the induction of hypnosis, brain waves slow down from the normal waking state (alpha waves) to a deeper state of relaxation (theta waves). Theta waves are commonly associated with deep relaxation, light sleep, and meditative states, and they are often observed in individuals who are highly absorbed in a task or suggestion. This brain wave activity contributes to the mental and emotional benefits of hypnosis, such as stress reduction, enhanced suggestibility, and therapeutic change.

3. Cognitive and Mental Changes

During hypnosis, the individual experiences various cognitive and mental changes that distinguish the hypnotic state from normal wakefulness. These changes include alterations in perception, memory, emotional processing, and attention. The person's mental processes become more flexible, allowing for the potential to address issues such as phobias, habits, and emotional blocks.

Key Cognitive and Mental Changes Include:

- *Focused Attention and Concentration*: One of the defining characteristics of hypnosis is the intense focus on a specific suggestion, image, or thought. The individual becomes highly concentrated on the hypnotist's words or the task at hand, allowing them to tune out external distractions and even internal distractions such as worries or self-judgments. This heightened focus is essential for the effectiveness of therapeutic hypnosis, such as in overcoming bad habits or changing deep-seated beliefs.

- *Heightened Suggestibility:* During hypnosis, the subconscious mind becomes more open and receptive to suggestions. This heightened suggestibility allows the hypnotist to introduce ideas, behaviors, or beliefs that the person may adopt more readily than in a normal state of consciousness. Suggestions given during hypnosis can lead to changes in perception, emotions, habits, or even physical sensations. For example, people under hypnosis may experience temporary pain relief or altered sensory experiences, such as feeling a hand warmer or cooler than usual.

- *Altered Memory and Perception:* Hypnosis can also affect memory and perception. For instance, under hypnosis, individuals may recall forgotten memories or experience vivid visualizations of events from the past. In some therapeutic applications, hypnosis can help a person access repressed memories or change how they view traumatic experiences. However, this process can also make people more susceptible to memory distortion, so hypnosis must be used carefully in therapeutic settings.

- *Emotional Shifts:* Hypnosis can bring about changes in how a person feels or reacts emotionally. For example, someone with a fear of flying may undergo hypnosis to reduce anxiety, making them feel more relaxed and comfortable when boarding a plane. Emotional shifts can also involve reducing stress, enhancing self-confidence, or overcoming limiting beliefs.

- *Dissociation:* Hypnosis often induces a form of dissociation, where a person feels detached from their surroundings or from certain parts of themselves. This detachment can help people reframe emotional experiences or perceptions. For instance, someone who has experienced trauma may temporarily dissociate from painful memories during hypnosis, allowing them to process those memories more effectively later on.

4. The Deepening of the Hypnotic State

Hypnosis is often described as occurring in different "depths," with the person experiencing varying levels of relaxation and suggestibility. The process of deepening the hypnotic state allows for a more profound influence on the subconscious mind.

Techniques to Deepen the Hypnotic State:

- *Progressive Relaxation:* The hypnotist may guide the person to relax progressively, focusing on relaxing each part of the body, from the feet up to the head, to induce a deeper state of calm and relaxation.
- *Imagery and Visualization:* Using vivid imagery, such as imagining descending a staircase or walking through a peaceful garden, can further deepen the hypnotic state and increase focus.
- *Counting or Deep Breathing:* Techniques like counting backward or practicing deep breathing help guide the person into a deeper state of hypnosis by encouraging relaxation and reinforcing focus.

The deeper the hypnotic state, the more susceptible a person may be to the suggestions given, allowing for profound therapeutic effects.

The hypnotic state is a unique experience that involves significant changes in both the mind and body. From physiological alterations such as reduced heart rate and muscle relaxation to profound changes in brain activity and cognitive processes, hypnosis is a complex and dynamic process. These changes allow hypnosis to be an effective tool for therapeutic purposes, such as pain management, behavior modification, and emotional healing. Understanding what happens during hypnosis gives us a clearer picture of its potential and highlights its versatility as a tool for self-improvement and well-being.

Induction and Deepening: Understanding How to Guide Someone into a Hypnotic State

Hypnosis is a skill that involves guiding someone into a deeply focused and relaxed state where they become highly suggestible to positive changes. The process of hypnotizing someone typically begins with an induction, which is a series of techniques used to bring the individual into a hypnotic state. Once the person has entered this initial relaxed state, further techniques can be employed to deepen the experience, making them even more focused and receptive to suggestions.

In this section, we will explore the different stages of induction, how to guide someone into hypnosis, and how to deepen the hypnotic state to maximize the effects.

1. *Understanding Induction*

Induction is the initial phase of hypnosis where the individual is guided from their usual waking state into a state of heightened suggestibility. During this phase, the goal is to induce relaxation and focused attention so the person's mind becomes open to suggestion.

Key Elements of Hypnotic Induction:

- *Relaxation:* The individual must feel physically and mentally relaxed. Hypnosis cannot occur effectively unless the person is relaxed enough to allow their subconscious mind to be more receptive.
- *Focused Attention:* Hypnosis involves directing the person's attention inward, away from the external environment. Focusing on a single thought, image, or sensation allows the individual to become

absorbed in the experience.

There are various methods for inducing hypnosis, and the approach may vary depending on the person's susceptibility and preferences. Common induction techniques include:

2. Common Induction Techniques

1. Progressive Relaxation:

Progressive relaxation is one of the most widely used methods of induction. It involves guiding the individual to progressively relax their muscles, starting from the toes and moving upward to the head.

How It Works:

- Begin by having the person sit or lie comfortably in a relaxed position.
- Ask them to focus on their breathing and take slow, deep breaths.
- Guide them to relax their toes, feet, legs, and then move upwards, directing their attention to each part of their body. Encourage them to notice any tension in their muscles and imagine that tension melting away.
- As the person progresses through their body, they should begin to feel a sense of deep relaxation spreading throughout their body.

Why It's Effective:

- Progressive relaxation works because it helps the person's body relax, which in turn helps their mind to relax.
- By focusing on one part of the body at a time, the individual can release physical tension and shift attention away from distractions, facilitating the entry into a hypnotic state.

2. Eye Fixation Induction:

Eye fixation induction relies on the individual's ability to focus their attention on a single point or object. This method is based on the principle that sustained focus helps induce a state of relaxation and concentration.

How It Works:

- Ask the person to sit comfortably and focus on a specific point in front of them, such as a spot on the wall or a small object (e.g., a pen or your finger).
- Encourage them to continue focusing on the object while you provide verbal suggestions. For example, you might say, "With every blink, you feel more relaxed."
- As the person focuses on the object, their attention becomes more absorbed in the process, and their mind starts to quiet down, allowing them to enter a relaxed, hypnotic state.

Why It's Effective:

- Eye fixation takes advantage of the mind-body connection. Focusing on an object causes the individual to narrow their attention, reducing distractions and promoting a sense of calm and concentration.

3. Breathing Techniques:
Breathing techniques are often used in combination with other induction methods to help induce relaxation and reduce mental chatter.
How It Works:

- Guide the person to take slow, deep breaths, inhaling through their nose and exhaling through their mouth.
- Encourage them to focus on the sensation of their breath, perhaps counting the breaths or imagining each breath as a wave that helps them become more relaxed.
- You may also suggest that with each exhalation, they release tension from their body, becoming more relaxed with each breath.

Why It's Effective:

- Deep breathing activates the parasympathetic nervous system, which is responsible for the body's relaxation response. Slow, deep breaths can help lower the heart rate and calm the mind, making it easier to enter a hypnotic state.

4. Visualization and Imagery:
Visualization is a powerful method that involves guiding the person to imagine a peaceful, relaxing scene. This technique is based on the idea that mental imagery can influence physical and emotional states.
How It Works:

- Ask the person to close their eyes and imagine a peaceful environment, such as a beach, a forest, or a quiet garden.
- Guide them to use all their senses to experience the scene. For example, suggest that they feel the warmth of the sun, hear the sound of waves or birds, and smell the fresh air.
- As they immerse themselves in the imagery, they will naturally feel more relaxed and focused, making it easier to enter a hypnotic state.

Why It's Effective:

- Engaging the imagination helps distract the person from external stimuli and promotes deep relaxation.
- By immersing them in a vivid, peaceful environment, the individual's mind shifts into a more receptive state, making it easier to access the subconscious.

3. Deepening the Hypnotic State

Once the person is in a relaxed, focused state, the next step is to deepen the hypnotic experience. This stage involves guiding the person into an even deeper level of hypnosis, which enhances the effectiveness of suggestions and therapeutic interventions.
Key Techniques for Deepening Hypnosis:
1. Counting Down:
One of the most common methods of deepening hypnosis is counting down from a specific number, typically from 10 or 20. This technique plays on the natural human tendency to relax and let go of conscious control as the numbers decrease.

How It Works:

- Once the person is relaxed, begin counting down slowly, suggesting that with each number, they will become more deeply relaxed and focused.
- For example, you could say, "With each number I count, you'll go deeper and deeper into relaxation. Ten... feeling more relaxed, Nine... sinking deeper, Eight... even more relaxed."

Why It's Effective:

- Counting creates a rhythm and offers a sense of progression, encouraging the person to let go more and more with each number. It reinforces the process of deepening the hypnotic state and promotes further relaxation.

2. Deepening with Imagery:

Imagery can also be used to deepen the hypnotic state. The idea is to have the person imagine descending into a deeper level of relaxation, which allows their mind to enter a more receptive state.

How It Works:

- Ask the individual to imagine descending a staircase, sinking deeper with each step. You can suggest that with every step they take, they feel more relaxed and comfortable.
- You might say, "With every step, you are going deeper into relaxation. Ten steps down, and with each one, you feel more peaceful, more calm, more open."

Why It's Effective:

- Imagery and visualization deepen the hypnotic experience by giving the person a vivid mental image to focus on. This deepens their absorption in the experience and heightens their suggestibility.

3. Physical Relaxation Cues:

Another method for deepening hypnosis is to suggest additional physical relaxation cues, such as feeling more warmth, heaviness, or lightness in certain parts of the body. These cues encourage the person to become more attuned to their body's sensations, which in turn enhances relaxation.

How It Works:

- Once the person is in a relaxed state, suggest that their body is becoming heavier or lighter, or that certain areas (such as their hands or feet) are becoming warm and comfortable.
- For example, you could say, "Your hands are becoming warm and heavy, and your body feels more relaxed with every breath you take."

Why It's Effective:

- Suggesting physical sensations helps anchor the person's focus in their body, further increasing relaxation. These physical sensations also serve as reminders that they are entering a deeper state of hypnosis.

4. Ensuring Deep Focus and Suggestibility

As the person's relaxation deepens, their ability to focus and be receptive to suggestions increases. At this point, you can begin to introduce positive suggestions or therapeutic interventions. The depth of hypnosis at this stage allows for greater effectiveness in addressing issues like pain, anxiety, bad habits, or stress.

Induction and deepening are critical components in the process of hypnosis. Induction involves guiding the person into a relaxed, focused state, while deepening techniques enhance the effectiveness of the hypnotic experience. By using various methods such as progressive relaxation, eye fixation, breathing techniques, and visualization, the hypnotist can help the individual achieve a profound state of focus and suggestibility. Deepening the hypnotic state further enhances the power of suggestions, making it a valuable tool for therapeutic change, personal growth, and self-improvement.

Chapter 4: Building Rapport and Trust

The Importance of Trust

When it comes to hypnosis, trust is one of the most crucial elements for success. The hypnotic process involves the subject's willingness to relax deeply, follow instructions, and accept suggestions. Without trust in the hypnotist, these actions become significantly more difficult, and the effectiveness of hypnosis is greatly diminished. Building a trusting relationship with your subject is the foundation upon which all successful hypnosis is built.

In this section, we will explore why trust is essential in hypnosis and offer practical steps on how to establish and nurture that trust. This chapter will provide insights into how you, as a hypnotist, can create a safe, supportive, and confident environment that encourages cooperation from the subject, helping them enter and remain in the hypnotic state.

1. Why Trust Is Essential in Hypnosis

Hypnosis is a process that requires full cooperation from the subject. This cooperation is most easily achieved when the person feels safe, comfortable, and confident in the hypnotist's abilities. Trust is integral for several reasons:

- *Relaxation and Focus:* In order to enter a deep state of hypnosis, the subject must feel completely relaxed. If they are anxious or unsure about the process, they may have difficulty letting go of their control and relaxing deeply. Trust in the hypnotist creates the comfort needed for the subject to feel secure enough to enter hypnosis.

- *Willingness to Follow Suggestions:* Hypnosis works by making the subconscious mind more open to suggestions. The subject must be willing to accept these suggestions in order for hypnosis to be effective. Trust in the hypnotist increases the subject's openness to suggestions, ensuring that the desired changes (e.g., breaking a bad habit, overcoming a fear) are more likely to take place.

- *Sense of Safety:* The hypnotic state is a vulnerable one for many people, as they are placing their full attention and control into the hands of the hypnotist. Trust ensures that the subject feels safe during the process and is more likely to cooperate.
- *Effective Communication:* Good communication is critical in hypnosis. A trusting relationship allows for better communication between the hypnotist and the subject, ensuring that the hypnotist's suggestions are clear, and the subject's responses and feedback are accurately interpreted.

2. How to Build Trust with Your Subject

Building trust doesn't happen instantly—it requires time, effort, and attention. However, the process can be accelerated by following certain principles that foster a positive, respectful relationship with the subject. Here are some strategies to help you build trust as a hypnotist:

1. Be Professional and Respectful

From the moment you meet your subject, it's important to convey professionalism and respect. Demonstrating that you are someone they can trust starts with showing genuine care and interest in their well-being.

- *Establish Clear Boundaries:* Set professional boundaries and make it clear that you are there to help them achieve their goals. Be upfront about what hypnosis is, how it works, and what they can expect from the session.
- *Respect Their Comfort Levels*: Always respect the subject's personal boundaries. Some people may feel uncomfortable with certain aspects of hypnosis, such as eye fixation or touch. Make sure to ask for permission and be flexible in your approach.
- *Be Transparent:* Let your subject know what the process involves, and explain the techniques you'll use in clear, simple language. Transparency about your methods fosters trust and reduces anxiety.

2. Show Empathy and Understanding

Empathy is key in building rapport. When you show that you truly understand and care about the subject's concerns, they are more likely to trust you.

- *Active Listening:* Listen carefully to the subject's needs and concerns. Ask open-ended questions and show that you are attentive to their responses. This will make the person feel heard and valued.
- *Non-Judgmental Attitude:* Approach each subject without judgment. Let them know that you accept and support them, no matter what issues they wish to address. A non-judgmental attitude will help create an atmosphere of trust and openness.
- *Acknowledge Their Fears:* If the subject expresses fear or skepticism about hypnosis, validate those feelings and reassure them. Explain that their experience is unique, and that you will work at a pace that feels comfortable for them.

3. Be Confident and Calm

Confidence is contagious. If you demonstrate self-assurance and composure throughout the hypnosis process, your subject is more likely to feel comfortable and trust you.

- *Confidence in Your Abilities*: If you are confident in your knowledge and ability to guide the subject through the process, your subject will feel reassured that they are in safe hands. This is especially important when you are first building a relationship with a new subject.
- *Maintain Calmness:* A calm demeanor will help put your subject at ease. If they see that you are composed and relaxed, it will help them feel more confident in the process. Anxiety is contagious, so your own sense of calm will naturally influence your subject's state of mind.
- *Lead with Positive Assurance:* Throughout the process, use positive, assuring language to make the subject feel secure. For example, phrases like, "You are doing great," or "You are safe and in control," can help boost the subject's confidence and trust in you.

4. Establish Clear Communication

Good communication is essential to building trust. In order for hypnosis to be effective, you must ensure that your subject understands the process and feels comfortable asking questions if they need clarification.

- *Explain the Process*: Clearly explain what will happen during the session. Let the subject know how long it will take, what techniques you will use, and what they should expect at each stage of the process.
- *Check for Understanding*: Periodically check in with your subject to ensure they understand what is happening. Ask if they are comfortable and if they have any questions.
- *Encourage Feedback:* Invite the subject to provide feedback throughout the session. Ask if they are feeling comfortable, if something is not working, or if they feel any discomfort. This will not only help you adjust the process to suit their needs but also build trust by showing that their comfort and well-being are your priority.

5. Build a Comfortable Environment

A comfortable, safe environment is essential for building trust. People are less likely to open up and relax if they are in an uncomfortable or distracting setting.

- *Create a Relaxing Atmosphere:* Set up a calm, quiet space free from distractions. Use soft lighting, comfortable seating, and a relaxing ambiance to promote a sense of peace.
- *Provide Comfort and Reassurance*: Ensure that your subject feels physically comfortable, whether that means adjusting the seating, offering a blanket, or providing an option to lie down. A person who is comfortable in their surroundings is more likely to trust you and relax into the hypnotic state.
- *Be Sensitive to Their Needs*: Check in with your subject to ensure they are not experiencing discomfort. If they need a break, more time, or a change in technique, be flexible and responsive to their needs.

3. Establishing Trust Over Time

Building trust does not end with a single session. While you can establish a strong initial rapport, trust grows over time with consistency and care.

- *Follow Through on Commitments*: Always follow through on any commitments or promises you make. If you say you will work on a specific issue or technique, ensure that you do so. Reliability fosters trust.
- *Respect Their Progress*: Acknowledge and celebrate small victories with the subject. If they've made progress or have achieved a breakthrough, validate their experience. Positive reinforcement strengthens the relationship and keeps the subject engaged in the process.
- *Be Patient*: Trust takes time to develop, especially if the subject has had prior negative experiences with hypnosis or if they are naturally skeptical. Be patient, and allow them to move at their own pace.

Building trust is the cornerstone of effective hypnosis. Without trust, the subject will have difficulty relaxing, following suggestions, and achieving the desired results. By maintaining professionalism, showing empathy, being confident and calm, and establishing clear communication, you can foster a trusting relationship with your subject. This trust is essential not only for successful hypnosis but also for creating a safe and supportive environment where meaningful change can occur.

Effective Communication Techniques: Verbal and Non-Verbal Cues to Create Rapport

Effective communication is one of the most important aspects of building trust and rapport in any relationship, including that of a hypnotist and their subject. In hypnosis, the success of the session often depends on how well the hypnotist can communicate with the subject, both verbally and non-verbally. Rapport, the bond of mutual respect and understanding, plays a crucial role in facilitating a relaxed, open environment where the subject can fully engage with the hypnotic process.

This section will explore verbal and non-verbal communication techniques that can help you build rapport, enhance the effectiveness of hypnosis, and ensure the subject feels safe, comfortable, and willing to follow your guidance.

1. Verbal Communication Techniques

Verbal communication involves the words you use, the tone of voice, and how you structure your suggestions. It's not just about the content of what you say, but how it is said. The goal is to make the subject feel understood, supported, and relaxed throughout the process.

1.1. Use of Positive and Reassuring Language

In hypnosis, language is a tool that can either relax or cause anxiety. Positive, calm, and reassuring words are essential for creating an atmosphere of trust and relaxation.

- *Focus on Positive Suggestions*: Use affirming and empowering language. Instead of saying, "You won't feel anxious," reframe it with a positive approach like, "You will feel calm and at ease." Positive phrasing helps the subconscious mind respond in a constructive way.
- *Provide Reassurance*: Offer words that comfort and assure the subject that they are in control, such as "You are safe," "You can go as deep as you wish," or "You will always be aware of what's happening."
- *Use Soothing and Calming Tone*: The tone in which you speak is just as important as the words themselves. Speak in a slow, steady, and soft tone to help induce relaxation. Avoid speaking too quickly, as this can create tension and anxiety.
- *Use of Simple, Clear Language*: Speak in a simple and clear manner, especially when giving instructions. Too many complex or abstract terms may confuse the subject and disrupt the hypnotic process.

1.2. Pacing and Leading

Pacing and leading is a technique used to build rapport by matching and guiding the subject's experience. It's about creating harmony in the communication and then gradually guiding the subject towards the desired state.

- *Pacing*: Start by matching the subject's current state—both physically and emotionally. If they seem tense, acknowledge their tension with empathetic statements like, "I can sense that you're feeling a bit nervous right now." This establishes a sense of understanding and empathy.
- *Leading*: Once you've established rapport by pacing their state, you can begin to lead them toward a relaxed or hypnotic state. For example, after acknowledging their tension, you might guide them with a statement like, "And as you take a deep breath in and let it out, you may begin to feel more relaxed." By leading them through small steps, you help them transition into a deeper state of hypnosis.
- *Gradual Progression*: Use pacing and leading to guide the subject through various stages of relaxation or trance. Pacing helps to establish trust, while leading is essential for guiding them toward deeper hypnotic states.

1.3. Embedded Suggestions

Embedded suggestions are a subtle and powerful communication technique where suggestions are woven into conversational language. This method allows the subject to absorb suggestions without feeling overwhelmed or coerced.

- *Use of Conversational Phrasing*: Instead of directly telling someone to do something, you might embed the suggestion within a broader sentence. For example, "As you sit there, you might find yourself feeling more relaxed, and you might notice how easy it is to let go of any tension."
- *Indirect Suggestions*: Using language that implies a possibility rather than a command can also be very effective. For example, saying, "You could begin to feel more relaxed as your body becomes heavier," is less direct and more flexible, allowing the subconscious mind to accept the suggestion more easily.

2. Non-Verbal Communication Techniques

Non-verbal cues are just as important—if not more so—than verbal communication when it comes to building rapport. Non-verbal communication includes your body language, facial expressions, and even how you physically position yourself during the session. These cues can help convey warmth, empathy, and attentiveness, fostering trust and comfort.

2.1. Body Language and Posture

Your posture and body language send powerful signals about your confidence, openness, and attentiveness. Being mindful of how you carry yourself during a hypnosis session can significantly enhance your ability to build rapport with your subject.

- *Open and Relaxed Posture:* Maintain an open and non-threatening posture. Avoid crossing your arms, as this can appear defensive. Instead, keep your body relaxed, with your arms at your sides or hands resting comfortably in front of you. A relaxed posture communicates calmness and invites the subject to relax as well.
- *Leaning In*: Slightly leaning toward the subject during conversation (without invading their personal space) can signal attentiveness and interest. This non-verbal cue helps the subject feel that they have your full attention.
- *Mirroring the Subject*: Subtly mirroring the subject's body language is a powerful technique to build rapport. If the subject is sitting with their hands resting calmly, try adopting a similar position. This mirroring can create a subconscious connection and increase the subject's comfort level.

2.2. Facial Expressions

Facial expressions convey empathy, understanding, and openness. Your face should reflect your attentiveness and support for the subject's process.

- *Smiling Gently*: A gentle, warm smile can instantly put a person at ease and create a sense of connection. However, avoid over-smiling, as it can seem insincere or forced.
- *Maintain Eye Contact:* Use appropriate eye contact to convey interest

and attentiveness. However, avoid staring aggressively or intensely, as this can be intimidating. Instead, aim for natural, soft eye contact, which can help the subject feel seen and understood.

- *Relaxed Face:* Keep your facial muscles relaxed and avoid showing tension. A tense or stiff face can make the subject feel uncomfortable or anxious. A calm, relaxed expression will mirror the calm atmosphere you wish to create.

2.3. Voice and Breathing Cues

While your words matter, the way you deliver them is equally important. Your voice's tone, pace, and volume can enhance relaxation or create tension.

- *Pacing Your Speech:* As you guide the subject into a relaxed state, adjust your speech rate. Slow down your speech slightly, using pauses between phrases to allow the subject to process the information. This slower pace mimics the relaxed, tranquil state you are guiding them into.

- *Breathing with the Subject*: A powerful way to create a deep connection is by mirroring the subject's breathing patterns. If they are taking slow, deep breaths, match their rhythm. Synchronizing your breathing with theirs can help induce a deeper sense of calm, as people naturally sync their breathing with others when they feel comfortable and connected.

2.4. Touch and Proximity

Touch and proximity can be powerful tools in communication, but they must always be used with caution, sensitivity, and respect for personal boundaries.

- *Non-Invasive Touch*: If appropriate and agreed upon, a light touch on the arm or shoulder can help convey support and warmth. However, always ask for permission first and respect the subject's preferences.

- *Respecting Personal Space*: Pay attention to the subject's comfort level when it comes to proximity. Some people may feel uneasy if you get too close. Respecting their personal space allows them to feel more at ease and less anxious.

3. Creating a Harmonious Communication Flow

In order to create effective rapport, both verbal and non-verbal communication must work in harmony. Your words, body language, and energy should all align to convey a sense of calm, openness, and empathy.

- *Consistency Between Verbal and Non-Verbal Cues:* Ensure that your words match your body language. If you are giving calming instructions but appear tense, the subject may feel confused or uncomfortable. Aligning your verbal cues with non-verbal signals creates consistency and reinforces the trust-building process.
- *Be Attentive to the Subject's Cues*: Pay attention to the subject's verbal and non-verbal cues. If they seem tense or uneasy, adjust your approach accordingly. If they are responding positively, deepen the rapport by continuing with what seems to be working.

Effective communication is essential to building rapport and trust with your subject in hypnosis. By using positive language, pacing and leading, and embedding suggestions, you can create an open and receptive atmosphere. Non-verbal cues such as body language, facial expressions, voice tone, and proximity also play a significant role in enhancing communication and making the subject feel comfortable and safe. Together, verbal and non-verbal techniques work to foster a trusting relationship, facilitating a deeper and more effective hypnotic experience.

Establishing a Safe Environment: Ensuring Your Subject Feels Comfortable and Safe

Creating a safe and comfortable environment is essential for successful hypnosis. When a subject feels physically and emotionally safe, they are more likely to relax deeply, trust you, and be receptive to the process. A sense of safety allows the mind to open up and facilitates the hypnotic experience, making it easier for the subject to enter a trance state.

This section will explore practical strategies for establishing a safe environment, both physically and psychologically, ensuring that your subject feels at ease throughout the session.

1. Physical Safety and Comfort

The physical environment in which hypnosis takes place plays a vital role in fostering a sense of safety. When your subject feels physically comfortable, they are more likely to relax and be open to the process.

1.1. Choosing a Quiet, Distraction-Free Space

The environment should be quiet and free from distractions. Noise, interruptions, or a chaotic setting can interfere with the subject's ability to focus and enter a trance. Select a room that is comfortable, private, and conducive to relaxation. Here's how you can set up the space:

- *Minimize Distractions:* Ensure that the space is free from external disturbances, such as loud noises, phones ringing, or people entering the room. A quiet environment helps the subject stay focused and relaxed.
- *Comfortable Temperature:* Ensure the room temperature is comfortable, neither too hot nor too cold. An uncomfortable temperature can distract the subject and prevent them from fully relaxing.
- *Comfortable Seating or Lying Arrangement*: Whether your subject is sitting or lying down, make sure the seating arrangement is comfortable. Provide pillows, blankets, or support as needed. Comfort allows the body to relax, which is essential for entering a hypnotic state.

1.2. Proper Lighting

Lighting can have a significant impact on the atmosphere of the room. A harsh, bright light can create tension or make the environment feel cold or sterile. Instead:

- *Soft, Indirect Lighting*: Use soft, ambient lighting or dimmed lights. This creates a calming atmosphere that helps the subject feel relaxed and comfortable.

- *Avoid Overhead Fluorescent Lights:* If possible, avoid using overhead fluorescent lights, as they can be harsh and unappealing. Opt for lamps with soft, warm light or candles (safely placed).

1.3. Comfortable Seating Position

When the subject is comfortable in their physical position, they can relax their body, which is critical for entering hypnosis.

- *Provide Relaxing Seating:* If the subject is sitting, ensure that the chair or seating option is comfortable and supportive. If they are lying down, ensure the surface is supportive enough to prevent discomfort.
- *Offer Pillows or Cushions:* Offer pillows or cushions to help them maintain a comfortable posture. Small adjustments, such as supporting their head, neck, or back, can improve their comfort level.
- *Positioning for Relaxation:* For many people, sitting or lying down with their arms and legs uncrossed is ideal, as this helps reduce physical tension. Encourage the subject to let go of any tension in their body to facilitate relaxation.

1.4. Personal Comfort Items

Allow the subject to bring personal items or comfort tools that help them feel more at ease, such as:

- *Blankets:* Some people may feel more secure or cozy with a blanket. If the subject requests one, be sure to provide it.
- *Comfortable Clothing:* Encourage the subject to wear comfortable clothing or remove any tight or restrictive clothing that could distract from the session.
- *Aromatherapy:* For some individuals, scents such as lavender, chamomile, or sandalwood can be calming. You could consider using essential oils or diffusers to enhance the ambiance.

2. Emotional and Psychological Safety

While physical comfort is essential, emotional and psychological safety is just as crucial. The subject must feel that they can trust you, and that they are in a space where their emotional well-being is respected. This is achieved by creating a nurturing, supportive, and empathetic environment.

2.1. Building Trust and Rapport

Before hypnosis begins, you must establish a trusting relationship with the subject. If they feel emotionally safe with you, they will be more willing to let go and fully engage in the hypnotic process.

- *Be Transparent and Clear:* Clearly explain what hypnosis is and what they can expect. Transparency helps demystify the process, reducing any fears or uncertainties they might have. Reassure them that they are always in control.
- *Show Empathy and Understanding:* Acknowledge any concerns the subject may have. For example, if they feel nervous or skeptical, listen to their feelings and validate them. A non-judgmental attitude fosters a sense of emotional safety.
- *Create a Positive First Impression*: The first few moments of the session set the tone for the entire experience. Greet the subject with warmth and make sure they feel welcomed and comfortable right from the beginning.

2.2. Ensure Consent and Comfort with the Process

Consent is a key component of emotional safety. The subject must feel comfortable with each aspect of the process and be able to withdraw at any time.

- *Gain Explicit Consent:* Ensure that the subject understands what the hypnosis session involves. Ask if they are comfortable proceeding and explain any techniques you will use (such as touch, breathing exercises, or eye fixation).
- *Allow for Flexibility:* Let the subject know they can stop the session at any time. Reassure them that if they feel uncomfortable or uncertain,

they can open their eyes and come out of the trance.

- *Check-In During the Session:* Regularly check in with the subject to see if they are comfortable and at ease. Phrases like, "How are you feeling right now?" or "Are you comfortable with what we're doing so far?" help ensure they feel heard and safe.

2.3. Respect Boundaries

It's important to respect the subject's physical and emotional boundaries throughout the process. Everyone has different comfort levels when it comes to hypnosis, and it's essential to honor these limits.

- *Non-Invasive Techniques:* If the hypnosis session involves touch (e.g., placing your hand on the subject's shoulder or wrist), always ask for permission first. Use gentle, non-invasive techniques, and make sure the subject is comfortable with them.
- *Physical Proximity*: Be mindful of the space between you and your subject. Some people may feel uncomfortable if you stand too close, while others may need physical reassurance to feel at ease.
- *Avoid Sensitive Topics:* If a subject has indicated that they have concerns about certain issues (such as trauma, phobias, or past experiences), ensure that you are not inadvertently bringing them up without their permission. Always respect their emotional boundaries.

2.4. Offer Reassurance and Support

At any point during the hypnosis session, if the subject shows signs of anxiety or discomfort, it's essential to offer reassurance and support. For instance, if they seem confused or uneasy, remind them that they are safe and that they can take their time to relax.

- *Reassure with Confidence:* Offer calming, positive statements like, "You are in a safe space, and you are in control of the process."
- *Use Gentle Touch (When Appropriate):* If appropriate and welcomed, a gentle hand on the shoulder or a soft touch can be comforting. However, always ask for permission and pay attention to how the

subject responds.

- *Provide a Comfortable Exit*: Let the subject know that they can come out of hypnosis whenever they wish. Giving them the power to end the session when needed fosters a sense of control and psychological safety.

3. Mental and Emotional Readiness

Before you begin the session, it's important to assess the subject's mental and emotional state. This will help you understand their needs and ensure that they are ready for hypnosis.

- *Assess Mental Readiness:* Some subjects may not be ready for hypnosis due to anxiety, stress, or other mental health concerns. Ensure they are in a calm and stable state before beginning.
- *Ask About Expectations:* Understanding the subject's goals and expectations helps to tailor the session to their needs. It also shows them that you care about their experience and are committed to helping them reach their objectives.

Creating a safe environment for hypnosis is not just about physical comfort, but also about emotional and psychological security. By ensuring that the space is quiet and comfortable, respecting the subject's boundaries, and fostering a trusting, empathetic relationship, you can establish an environment where the subject feels safe, supported, and ready to engage in the process. This sense of safety is key to making the hypnosis experience effective and empowering for the subject, allowing them to fully relax and open themselves up to the potential of change.

Chapter 5: Hypnotic Induction Techniques

Progressive Relaxation: A Step-by-Step Guide to the Most Common Induction Technique

Progressive relaxation is one of the most widely used and effective hypnotic induction techniques. It involves guiding the subject into a state of deep relaxation by progressively relaxing different parts of the body, typically starting from the toes and moving upwards towards the head. This method works by helping the subject become aware of the sensations in their body and letting go of tension, preparing them to enter a deeper state of hypnosis.

In this chapter, we will explore how to use progressive relaxation as an induction technique, providing you with a step-by-step guide to conducting it effectively.

1. Preparing the Subject for Induction

Before beginning the progressive relaxation induction, it's important to ensure that your subject is physically and mentally prepared for the process. Take the following steps:

- *Ensure Comfort:* Make sure the subject is seated or lying in a comfortable position. If they are lying down, make sure their body is well-supported with pillows or cushions. A relaxed posture will help facilitate the relaxation process.
- *Set the Environment:* As discussed in previous chapters, the room should be quiet, with soft lighting, and free from distractions. Adjust the temperature and ensure that the subject will be comfortable throughout the session.
- *Establish Rapport:* Take a few moments to build rapport and trust with the subject. A calm, soothing tone of voice and clear

instructions will help ease any potential tension or resistance.

- *Reassure the Subject:* Let them know that they are safe and that they can stop the process at any time if they wish. Reassure them that they will remain in control at all times.

2. The Progressive Relaxation Induction Technique: Step-by-Step

Step 1: Focus on Breathing

The first step in any relaxation process is to guide the subject's focus to their breath. Breathing is a natural way to begin reducing tension and focusing the mind.

- *Instructions*: Begin by asking the subject to take a slow, deep breath in through their nose, and then exhale gently through their mouth. Encourage them to continue breathing slowly and deeply, focusing on the rhythm of their breath.
- *Reassurance*: As they breathe, offer gentle reassurance: "With each breath, you're becoming more relaxed... deeper and deeper with every breath you take."

This process helps the subject shift their focus from external distractions to internal sensations, starting the relaxation process.

Step 2: Focus on the Feet and Legs

Start at the very base of the body, guiding the subject to relax their feet and legs.

- *Instructions*: Ask the subject to direct their attention to their feet. Instruct them to feel any tension or discomfort in their feet, then slowly release it, allowing their feet to become warm and heavy.
    - "Focus on your feet now... Feel the muscles in your feet and toes. Let them soften and relax... As you breathe out, release all the tension from your feet... Let them feel warm, heavy, and completely relaxed."
- *Progress*: Continue by guiding them to relax their lower legs (calves), knees, and thighs in the same manner. Encourage them to notice and

release any tension.

  - ○ "Now, move your attention to your calves... feel any tightness melting away. Allow your knees to soften... and your thighs to become heavy and relaxed."

Encourage slow, deliberate relaxation as they focus on these areas, helping them feel the gradual release of tension.

Step 3: Relax the Abdomen and Chest
Now that the subject's legs are relaxed, move up to the torso. This area often holds a significant amount of tension, so it's important to guide them carefully through the process.

- *Instructions*: Ask the subject to bring their awareness to their abdomen and chest. Instruct them to take a deep breath and feel their belly rise and fall. With each exhalation, they should allow the muscles in their abdomen and chest to relax.
  - ○ "Now bring your attention to your abdomen. With each breath you take, feel the muscles soften and relax. As you breathe out, imagine all the tension leaving your body, allowing your abdomen to become soft and loose."
  - ○ "Move your awareness now to your chest... with each exhalation, feel your chest gently open and relax. Let go of any tightness, allowing your chest to become warm and relaxed."

This helps the subject enter a deeper state of relaxation by releasing tension in the areas most often associated with stress and anxiety.

Step 4: Relax the Shoulders, Arms, and Hands
The shoulders and arms are common areas where tension can accumulate, so focus on relaxing these areas next.

- *Instructions*: Guide the subject to bring their awareness to their shoulders. Instruct them to let go of any tension in this area, imagining their shoulders becoming heavy and sinking down.
  - ○ "Now, bring your focus to your shoulders. Notice any

tension or tightness, and let it all go. Feel your shoulders become warm and heavy, letting them sink deeper into the surface beneath you."

- *Progressing Down the Arms*: Continue with the arms, asking them to relax their upper arms, elbows, lower arms, and hands.
    - "Now, move your attention to your arms, all the way down to your hands. Allow the muscles in your arms to loosen, and feel any tension draining out of your fingertips. Your arms are completely relaxed and heavy."

This step helps release built-up tension and encourages a sense of deep relaxation in the upper body.

Step 5: Relax the Neck, Face, and Head
The neck, face, and head are crucial areas that often hold subconscious tension. It is important to guide the subject through relaxation in these areas with care.

- *Instructions*: Ask the subject to focus on their neck, allowing the muscles to soften and relax.
    - "Now, bring your awareness to your neck. Let go of any tightness, and feel the muscles in your neck soften, releasing all the tension."
- *Face and Jaw Relaxation*: Direct their attention to their face, asking them to relax their jaw, forehead, and the muscles around the eyes.
    - "Move your focus to your face now... Let your jaw unclench, your lips soften, and your eyes feel relaxed. Feel your forehead smooth out, releasing any tension."
- *Complete Relaxation of the Head:* Finally, guide them to relax their scalp and the top of their head.
    - "Now, relax your scalp and the top of your head. Feel the muscles in your head soften and release any remaining tension, letting go completely."

This stage is vital for ensuring that the subject's entire body is relaxed and ready to enter a deep hypnotic state.

Step 6: Deepening the Relaxation
Once the subject's body is completely relaxed, you can deepen the hypnotic state by adding deepening techniques. This can help them enter a more profound level of hypnosis.

- *Deepening Suggestions:* At this point, you can suggest that the subject feels even more relaxed with every breath, and that they are entering a deeper state of calm and stillness.
    - "With each breath, you go deeper into relaxation... With every sound you hear, you feel more and more at ease. Let yourself go deeper into the stillness and calm of your mind."

You may also use imagery to deepen the trance:

- *Visualization*: "Imagine you are descending a staircase, with each step taking you deeper into a peaceful, calm state. With each step, your body relaxes more deeply, and your mind becomes even more peaceful."

3. Completion and Transition into Hypnosis
Once the subject has reached a relaxed and deep state, you can transition them into the therapeutic phase of hypnosis, whether that be suggestion work, regression, or other hypnotic techniques.

- *Induction Completion*: After the subject has relaxed completely, gently suggest that they are now ready to receive positive suggestions, or whatever the purpose of the hypnosis session may be.
    - "You are now in a deeply relaxed state, your body and mind fully at ease. You are ready to explore new ideas, make positive changes, and embrace deep transformation."

Progressive relaxation is a gentle and effective way to guide a subject into hypnosis. By slowly relaxing each part of the body and focusing on the sensations of calmness and heaviness, you help the subject let go of tension and move into a deeply relaxed state. This induction method works well for beginners and experienced subjects alike, as it builds a strong foundation of physical relaxation, paving the way for deeper exploration of the mind and greater success in therapeutic hypnosis. By following the steps outlined here and practicing regularly, you'll be able to lead your subjects into a relaxed state with confidence and ease.

Eye Fixation Method: Focusing Attention to Induce Trance

The Eye Fixation Method is another popular and effective hypnotic induction technique that uses the subject's natural ability to focus their attention to guide them into a trance. This method involves having the subject focus on a particular point or object, such as a light, a spot on the wall, or your hand, while encouraging them to relax deeply and allow their attention to narrow. As their eyes tire and their attention becomes more focused, they are gradually led into a deep state of hypnosis.

This technique is effective because it uses concentration and physical cues to promote relaxation and the eventual transition into a hypnotic trance. Below is a step-by-step guide on how to effectively perform the Eye Fixation Method.

1. Preparation and Environment

Before you begin the Eye Fixation induction, ensure the following:

- *Comfortable Setting:* Make sure your subject is seated in a comfortable position, either in a chair or lying down, where they can maintain a relaxed posture. You should aim to have them feel both physically and mentally at ease.
- *Lighting*: Ensure that the room is not too bright, but not too dark either. If using a light for fixation, it should be gentle and not too harsh. Dim lighting works best for this type of induction.
- *Avoid Distractions*: Minimize any distractions in the room, as this technique relies heavily on focus and attention. Ensure that the subject's eyes are free from discomfort.

2. The Eye Fixation Induction: Step-by-Step

Step 1: Introduce the Process and Set Expectations

Begin by explaining the process to the subject in a calm and reassuring voice, so they know what to expect.

- *Explanation*: "In just a moment, I will ask you to focus your attention on a point in front of you. As you do, you will begin to feel more and more relaxed with each breath, allowing your mind and body to become calm and peaceful."

Reassure them that they will remain in control and that the process will be completely safe. Let them know that their eyes may become tired or heavy, and that's a natural part of the process.

Step 2: Focus on the Object

Now, guide the subject to focus on an object or spot. Common choices include a light (such as a lamp or candle), a specific point on the wall, or your finger held a few inches from their eyes.

- *Instructions*: "Now, I want you to focus all of your attention on this spot or light. Notice the details of it, the shape, color, and texture. Keep your eyes focused on this point, and just allow your attention to narrow and become absorbed by it."

Encourage the subject to keep their focus on the object without straining their eyes, allowing them to simply observe it.

Step 3: Deepen Focus with Relaxation Suggestions

As the subject focuses their attention, give them suggestions to help them relax and become more absorbed in the process.

- *Instructions*: "With each breath you take, allow your eyes to become heavier and heavier, feeling more relaxed with every moment. The longer you focus on this point, the more relaxed you feel, and the more calm and peaceful your body and mind become."

You can also add:

- "As your eyes focus, you may notice them beginning to feel heavy, as if they are naturally closing... but keep them focused on that spot for as long as you can. The more relaxed you become, the easier it will be to keep your attention fixed."

Step 4: Encourage the Eyes to Close

As the subject continues to focus on the point, encourage them to allow their eyes to naturally begin to close, signaling the transition into deeper relaxation.

- *Suggestions*:
    - "The longer you focus on this spot, the more relaxed you feel, and the heavier your eyelids become... It's perfectly fine to let your eyes close when you feel they want to... and as they close, you'll go even deeper into relaxation."
    - "When your eyelids close, you'll find yourself feeling more relaxed and at ease. The more your eyes become relaxed, the more your body and mind will also relax."

At this point, the subject's eyelids may begin to flutter, and they may begin to blink more slowly or even close entirely. If they haven't closed yet, you can suggest:

- "Your eyes may want to close now, allowing you to drift even deeper into relaxation, letting go of any remaining tension."

Step 5: Deepen the Trance

Once the subject's eyes have closed, continue to deepen the trance by reinforcing relaxation and guiding them through physical or mental cues that encourage them to go deeper.

- *Breathing*: "Now that your eyes are closed, take a deep, slow breath in, and as you breathe out, feel yourself letting go of any tension. With each breath, you go deeper, feeling more relaxed and calm."
- *Progressive Relaxation*: If needed, you can begin using progressive relaxation techniques to guide the subject through further relaxation. For example:
    - "As your body relaxes, you may notice a feeling of warmth or heaviness spreading through your body... starting at your feet and moving up through your legs, your abdomen, chest, shoulders, arms, and neck. With every breath, you sink

deeper into this wonderful state of calm.”
- *Visual Imagery:* You can enhance the experience by guiding them to visualize a peaceful scene that deepens the trance:
  - ○ “Imagine now that you are walking down a staircase, with each step you take, you feel even more relaxed and at ease. Ten steps down, and with every step, you go deeper into calm, peaceful relaxation.”

Step 6: Final Deepening Suggestions
After deepening the trance, you can offer further suggestions for relaxation and focus. Reaffirm that they are in a safe and controlled environment.

- *Reassurance*: “As you continue to relax, you are in complete control. Your mind is clear, and you are free to relax as deeply as you need. All the stresses and worries are fading away as you focus deeply on the present moment.”

By offering continued suggestions of peace and calm, you'll help guide the subject into a deep trance, ready for therapeutic work or positive suggestion.

3. Transition into Therapeutic Work

Once the subject is in a relaxed and receptive state, you can transition into the specific goal of the hypnosis session, whether it's suggestion therapy, behavior change, pain relief, or another hypnotic process.

The Eye Fixation Method is an effective technique because it uses the natural human tendency to focus and concentrate. It allows the subject to direct their attention to a single point, which encourages relaxation and helps them let go of other distractions. Through this technique, the subject can easily transition from a focused state into a deeply relaxed and hypnotized state, ready for further exploration and therapeutic work.

By following these steps and practicing regularly, you can use eye fixation to induce hypnosis with confidence, guiding your subjects into a peaceful, relaxed state and helping them access the subconscious mind for healing, change, and growth.

Guided Visualization: Using Imagery to Deepen the Hypnotic State

Guided visualization, also known as *mental imagery* or *guided imagery,* is a powerful technique in hypnosis that uses vivid and soothing images to help the subject relax, focus, and enter a deeper hypnotic state. This technique leverages the mind's ability to create mental pictures and is especially effective in enhancing relaxation, helping the subject overcome stress, and reinforcing positive suggestions. Visualization is used in both induction and deepening phases of hypnosis, and it can be customized for various therapeutic goals, such as stress reduction, overcoming fears, or promoting healing.

In this chapter, we will explore how to use guided visualization to deepen the hypnotic state and help subjects access their subconscious mind for positive change.

1. Preparing the Subject for Guided Visualization

Before beginning a guided visualization, it is important to prepare the subject and the environment to ensure the process goes smoothly.

- *Comfortable Position:* Ensure the subject is in a comfortable seated or lying position. Their body should be relaxed, with no distractions.
- *Setting the Scene:* Dim the lights to create a calming atmosphere. If necessary, play soft, ambient music that helps the subject relax. Make sure the room is quiet and free from external disturbances.
- *Rapport and Reassurance*: Establish rapport with the subject and remind them that they are in control throughout the process. Let them know that if they feel uncomfortable at any point, they can stop the session.

2. The Guided Visualization Technique: Step-by-Step

Step 1: Inducing Relaxation

Before starting the visualization itself, you need to guide the subject into a state of deep relaxation. You can either use a progressive relaxation technique or another induction method to help the subject become more relaxed.

- *Instructions*: "Take a few deep breaths, slowly inhaling through your nose and exhaling through your mouth. With each breath, feel your body becoming more and more relaxed. Imagine any tension in your body melting away with each exhale."

Once the subject is relaxed, you can transition into the visualization portion of the session.

Step 2: Introduce the Visualization

The next step is to introduce the imagery to the subject. You can begin by suggesting they imagine a peaceful, calming scene. Be sure to use descriptive language to help the subject visualize clearly and vividly.

- *Instructions*: "Now, I want you to imagine yourself standing at the edge of a beautiful, tranquil beach. You can feel the soft, warm sand beneath your feet. The sun is shining gently, and you can hear the sound of the waves lapping against the shore. You feel safe, calm, and peaceful here, surrounded by the beauty of nature."

Encourage the subject to immerse themselves in the imagery. Use all the senses to paint a detailed picture, incorporating sounds, smells, sights, and sensations. The more detailed and sensory-rich the imagery, the more deeply the subject can engage with the visualization.

- *Sensory Details*: "As you stand on the beach, you can smell the salty air, feel the gentle breeze on your skin, and hear the rhythmic sound of the waves. You may even notice the warmth of the sun on your face, relaxing you even further."

Step 3: Deepening the Trance with Visualization

Now that the subject is focused on the imagery, you can deepen their relaxation and deepen the trance state by guiding them through a more immersive visualization.

- *Deeper Relaxation Suggestions:* "With each breath you take, you feel more deeply relaxed. As you breathe in, you inhale calmness and peace, and as you breathe out, you release any remaining tension or stress. The more you relax, the more deeply you can focus on the image of the beach, allowing yourself to become completely immersed in this peaceful place."
- *Progressing the Visualization:* To deepen the state, you can take the

subject through a progression of events within the visualization, guiding them deeper into relaxation or suggesting that they move through the scene. For example, you can have them walk down the beach, explore a calm forest, or sit by a peaceful stream.

- "Imagine now that you are walking along the shoreline, your feet sinking gently into the soft sand with each step. With every step you take, you feel even more relaxed, as though the earth itself is supporting you and helping you release any tension."
- "As you continue walking, you notice a comfortable lounge chair set up under a shade tree, inviting you to sit down and rest. You make your way over and sit in the chair, feeling the cool shade wrap around you. With each breath, you feel even more relaxed, more at peace."

By leading the subject through a series of calm, peaceful, and enjoyable experiences in the visualization, you help deepen the trance and encourage further relaxation.

Step 4: Engaging the Subconscious Mind

Once the subject is deeply relaxed and focused within the visualization, you can use this state to communicate with their subconscious mind. You can incorporate therapeutic suggestions, affirmations, or positive imagery.

- *Therapeutic Suggestions:* If the goal of the session is therapeutic (e.g., overcoming stress or fear), you can introduce positive suggestions during the visualization.
  - "As you sit in this peaceful place, you begin to feel a sense of confidence and calmness building inside you. You realize that you are capable of handling anything that comes your way, and you can carry this peace and strength with you wherever you go."
- *Positive Imagery*: You can guide the subject to imagine their desired outcome or goal within the visualization.
  - "Imagine now that a bright, glowing light is surrounding

you, filling you with warmth and energy. This light is filled with positivity, health, and strength. Let it bathe every part of your being, bringing healing, calmness, and a sense of well-being."

By guiding the subject to picture their goals and desired states within the visualization, you help reinforce those suggestions in a powerful, subconscious way.

Step 5: Reinforce Relaxation and Focus

As the subject becomes more absorbed in the visualization, continue reinforcing the deep relaxation and focus.

- *Reinforcing Relaxation:* "With each breath you take, you feel more deeply relaxed, more deeply connected to this peaceful scene. The more relaxed you are, the more focused you become. You are completely present in this moment, surrounded by calm and peace."
- *Focus on Inner Peace:* "This feeling of peace, calm, and relaxation is within you now. You can return to this place of tranquility anytime you need to feel calm and centered. Every time you think of this place, you will be able to instantly bring yourself into this peaceful state."

Step 6: Gradual Transition and Awakening

Once the therapeutic work or visualization phase is complete, guide the subject out of the hypnotic state gently and gradually.

- *Transition*: "In a moment, I will begin to count from one to five. With each number, you will begin to feel more awake and alert, bringing with you the calm and peace from this experience. One... slowly beginning to feel more aware of your surroundings. Two... becoming more and more alert. Three... feeling refreshed, calm, and positive. Four... bringing back all the peace and relaxation with you. Five... open your eyes, feeling completely awake, alert, and at ease."

Guided visualization is a powerful tool for deepening the hypnotic state because it engages the mind's creative faculties and encourages profound relaxation and focus. By guiding the subject through vivid, peaceful imagery, you create an environment where the subconscious mind is more open to positive suggestions and changes. Whether the purpose is stress reduction, behavioral change, or achieving a therapeutic goal, visualization can be a highly effective technique when used skillfully.

By practicing and refining your ability to guide your subject through these visualizations, you can help them achieve deep relaxation and use the power of their imagination to promote healing and personal growth.

Instant or Rapid Inductions: Techniques to Induce Hypnosis Quickly

Instant or rapid inductions are techniques used to induce a hypnotic state in a very short period of time, often within seconds to a few minutes. These methods are effective when you need to quickly guide someone into hypnosis, either for therapeutic purposes, stage hypnosis, or as part of a demonstration. Rapid inductions work by interrupting the subject's normal patterns of thought, using shock, surprise, or focused concentration to bypass the conscious mind and access the subconscious.

Below is an overview of popular techniques for inducing hypnosis quickly and effectively.

1. The Hand Drop Induction

One of the most common rapid induction techniques is the hand drop induction, which utilizes the natural tendency of the body to relax and surrender once it experiences a quick, focused suggestion. It's based on the principle that the subject's attention can be shifted instantly, and this shift helps induce hypnosis.

Step-by-Step:

- *Preparation*: Ask the subject to stand or sit comfortably in a relaxed position.
- *The Command*: "In a moment, I'm going to ask you to raise your right hand in front of you and focus on it. I want you to concentrate on the sensation in your hand, and as soon as you feel my hand touch yours, you will instantly enter a deep state of relaxation and hypnosis."

- *The Action:* As they focus on their hand, you quickly move to gently touch or grasp their hand, causing it to drop. The moment their hand begins to drop, you suggest, "As your hand drops, you will feel your whole body relax and drift into a deep state of hypnosis."
- *Induction Completion:* Use calming, deepening language as their hand drops and they relax. You can now guide them deeper into the trance using typical deepening techniques, like progressive relaxation or deepening suggestions.

The rapid drop of the hand creates a brief physical shock to the body, which immediately disrupts their normal conscious thinking and allows the subject to go into a relaxed, receptive state.

2. *The Confusion Induction*

The confusion induction is based on the principle of inducing cognitive overload. When the conscious mind becomes confused or distracted, it can quickly be overwhelmed and give way to the subconscious mind, which is more open to suggestions.

Step-by-Step:

- *Begin with Disorientation*: Start by giving the subject a series of rapidly shifting instructions or suggestions that don't make immediate sense, causing confusion. For example, you could say, "Take a deep breath in, but at the same time, notice your left hand going up while your right hand stays still... but focus on your breath, while you're noticing how heavy your right arm feels."
- *Interrupt Normal Thought:* Continue to give contradictory or rapid-fire commands. The goal is to make the conscious mind stop its usual processing to try to figure out what's happening. A mild state of confusion or overwhelm can set in.
- *Final Suggestion:* Once you feel the subject is beginning to mentally disconnect from the confusion, offer a strong hypnotic suggestion: "As you feel the confusion, your mind will let go, and you will relax completely, allowing yourself to drift into a deep, relaxed state of

hypnosis."

- *Deepening*: Once the subject is in a relaxed state, you can proceed with deepening techniques like progressive relaxation or imagery to deepen the trance.

The confusion induction works by disrupting the conscious thought process, creating a moment where the subject's mental focus becomes confused, allowing their subconscious mind to take over and enter a relaxed, hypnotic state.

3. The Arm Levitation Induction

The arm levitation induction is a quick and highly effective technique that uses the subject's unconscious physical responses to trigger the hypnotic state. It's often used in both therapeutic and stage hypnosis contexts.

Step-by-Step:

- *Initial Relaxation:* Begin by guiding the subject into a relaxed state using breathing techniques or progressive relaxation.
- *Suggest the Arm Movement:* "Now, I want you to relax your body and imagine that your right arm is becoming lighter, as if it's being gently lifted by an invisible string. Just allow it to start to float up."
- *Focused Attention:* As you suggest this, the subject will begin to notice their arm becoming lighter and may start to experience the sensation of their arm lifting. If necessary, you can guide them by gently placing a hand on their wrist or elbow to suggest movement.
- *Reinforcement*: "With every breath you take, your arm becomes lighter and lighter, and the moment it starts to rise, you will enter a deeper state of relaxation and focus. Just let it float up as you let go completely."
- *Complete the Induction*: When the subject's arm begins to rise (even slightly), you can suggest, "Now that your arm is rising, you are going deeper into relaxation and ready to enter hypnosis. Your body and mind are relaxed, and your unconscious is open to suggestion."

This method works quickly because the sensation of the arm rising creates a tangible and physical experience that distracts the conscious mind, allowing the subject to slip into a deeper, hypnotic state.

4. The Shock Induction (Startle Technique)

The shock induction is one of the fastest ways to induce hypnosis, especially in a stage hypnosis context. It involves a sudden, unexpected action (like a light touch or verbal cue) that disrupts the subject's normal state of alertness, causing an immediate drop into relaxation.

Step-by-Step:

- *Preparation*: Have the subject stand or sit in a comfortable position. It is helpful to have them relaxed and slightly focused but not yet fully hypnotized.
- *Unexpected Suggestion*: Speak quickly and use an unexpected or abrupt suggestion. For example, you might say, "And now, you're going to feel a deep sense of relaxation, but at the same time, I will clap my hands loudly."
- *Shock and Induction:* Just after you make the suggestion, you create the shock element—perhaps a sudden loud clap or a quick touch to their shoulder or hand. This startles the subject for a split second.
- *Reinforcement:* Immediately after the shock, you suggest: "That surprise has caused you to relax deeply, and you are now entering a state of deep hypnosis. Your body is relaxed, and your mind is calm and open to positive suggestions."

The shock induction works by startling the subject, interrupting their conscious thought processes and quickly redirecting their focus onto relaxation. The surprise element helps bypass the critical thinking of the conscious mind, allowing them to enter a trance state.

5. The "Now" Induction

This rapid induction involves an immediate, direct approach that aims to guide the subject into hypnosis with minimal delay. It uses direct verbal suggestions that shift the subject's awareness quickly.

Step-by-Step:

- *Direct Suggestion:* You begin by saying something like, "I'm going to count to three, and by the time I reach three, you will be in a deep state of hypnosis, deeply relaxed and focused. One, two, three—now."
- *Instant Relaxation*: As you say "now," give a strong suggestion that the subject immediately relaxes and enters a trance.
- *Deepening*: Once you've got the subject in a relaxed state, you can quickly deepen the trance using imagery, breathing, or other techniques.

The "Now" induction works well because it is direct and leaves no room for hesitation. The simple command combined with an immediate relaxation suggestion is enough to get the subject into a hypnotic state in a matter of seconds.

Instant and rapid inductions are useful tools for hypnotists who need to induce a trance quickly and efficiently. These techniques can be applied in various settings, including therapeutic environments, stage performances, or demonstrations. By using physical cues, surprise elements, and focused suggestions, you can guide a subject into a deep, relaxed state in a very short amount of time.

While rapid inductions may require practice to master, they are a highly effective way to bypass the conscious mind and allow the subject to access their subconscious for therapeutic change, relaxation, or performance.

Self-Hypnosis: How to Use Induction on Yourself

Self-hypnosis is the process of guiding yourself into a hypnotic state, allowing you to access your subconscious mind without the assistance of a hypnotist. It is a valuable tool for personal growth, relaxation, overcoming habits, and achieving therapeutic goals such as stress relief, improving confidence, or reducing anxiety. By learning how to induce hypnosis on yourself, you can harness the power of your subconscious mind to create positive changes in your life.

In this section, we will cover the steps involved in self-hypnosis, from preparation to induction and deepening, as well as how to use it effectively for various purposes.

1. Understanding Self-Hypnosis

Before you begin, it's important to understand the basics of self-hypnosis. Essentially, self-hypnosis is a form of deep relaxation and focused attention. In this state, your conscious mind relaxes, and your subconscious mind becomes more receptive to suggestions and positive affirmations.

Self-hypnosis involves:

- *Relaxation*: Entering a deeply relaxed state.
- *Focused Attention:* Focusing on a specific thought, image, or suggestion.
- *Suggestion*: Planting positive suggestions or affirmations into your subconscious mind.

2. Preparing for Self-Hypnosis

To practice self-hypnosis effectively, it's important to set the stage for success. Follow these initial steps to prepare yourself and your environment:

- *Choose a Quiet, Comfortable Place:* Find a calm, distraction-free environment. A comfortable chair or a soft spot on the floor where you can sit or lie down will work best.
- *Set a Goal*: Be clear about what you want to achieve with self-hypnosis. This could be relaxation, eliminating a negative habit, overcoming anxiety, or reinforcing positive behaviors.
- *Set an Intention for the Session*: Decide on the purpose of the session before you start. Whether you're looking to reduce stress, improve sleep, or change a behavior, having a clear intention helps guide your suggestions.
-

3. The Self-Hypnosis Induction Process

The goal of induction is to guide yourself into a relaxed, focused state, which makes the subconscious mind more accessible. Here's a step-by-step guide to self-hypnosis induction:

Step 1: Get Comfortable

- Sit or lie in a position that feels comfortable and relaxed.
- Close your eyes and begin to take slow, deep breaths.
  - *Example Suggestion*: "With every breath I take, I am becoming more and more relaxed."

Step 2: Progressive Relaxation

One of the most effective ways to enter a hypnotic state is through progressive relaxation. This technique involves tensing and relaxing each part of your body, helping to release physical tension and encourage relaxation.

- Start with your toes and work your way up the body, consciously relaxing each muscle group.
- *Example Suggestion:* "Starting with my toes, I relax every muscle, allowing the tension to melt away. Moving up to my feet, I feel them becoming heavy and relaxed. My legs relax completely, my torso becomes calm, my arms relax, and my head feels light."

Step 3: Focus Your Attention

Now, focus your attention on a single point or sensation, such as your breath, a specific part of your body, or a mental image. This focused attention helps deepen the trance and quiets the conscious mind.

- *Example Suggestion:* "I focus on the steady rhythm of my breathing, each breath bringing me deeper into relaxation. With every breath I take, I feel more and more peaceful and calm."

Alternatively, you can use visualization or guided imagery to help deepen your state of relaxation:

- Imagine yourself in a peaceful place, like a quiet beach or a beautiful garden. Picture all the details vividly, using all your senses (what you see, hear, smell, feel).

Step 4: Deepening the Trance
Once you've reached a state of relaxation, use deepening techniques to go further into trance. The deeper you go, the more accessible your subconscious mind becomes, allowing you to access more profound thoughts, memories, or emotional states.

- *Counting Down:* One popular technique is to count down from 10 to 1, with each number taking you deeper into relaxation.
  - *Example Suggestion:* "As I count backward from 10 to 1, I will go deeper into relaxation. Ten... feeling calm. Nine... deeper still. Eight... letting go of all tension. Seven... deeper with each breath. Six... more relaxed. Five... letting go completely. Four... peaceful and calm. Three... deeper. Two... almost there. One... deeply relaxed."
- *The Elevator Technique:* Imagine yourself in an elevator, and with each floor you descend, you become more deeply relaxed.
  - *Example Suggestion:* "I step into the elevator and press the button to descend. As the elevator moves down, I feel myself going deeper into relaxation. Each floor I pass takes me to a more peaceful, calm state."

4. Using Self-Hypnosis for Positive Change

Once you're in a deep hypnotic state, the subconscious mind becomes more receptive to suggestions. This is the time to introduce positive affirmations or suggestions to achieve your desired goal. The key is to make the suggestions simple, positive, and in the present tense.

Positive Suggestions Example:

- *For Relaxation:* "I am calm, at peace, and in control of my thoughts and emotions. I remain calm and relaxed in all situations."
- *For Overcoming Stress:* "I handle stressful situations with ease. My body and mind are relaxed and free from tension."
- *For Confidence:* "I am confident in myself and my abilities. I believe in

my strength to succeed in every situation."

- *For Smoking Cessation:* "I am a non-smoker. I no longer crave cigarettes. My body is healthy and free from addiction."

Visualization for Goal Achievement

Visualizing your desired outcome can also reinforce the effectiveness of self-hypnosis. Picture yourself successfully achieving your goal.

- *Example*: If you're using self-hypnosis to improve your confidence, visualize yourself confidently speaking or performing in front of others, feeling calm, composed, and successful.

5. Reinforcing Suggestions

Reinforce the positive suggestions you've made by repeating them during the session. The repetition of suggestions strengthens their impact on the subconscious mind.

- *Example Suggestion:* "I am calm, I am confident, I am in control. These positive changes are taking root within me and growing stronger every day."

You can also use *anchoring* techniques, where you associate a gesture (like tapping your fingers together) or a word with the positive state you're aiming for. This allows you to trigger the hypnotic state and positive feelings quickly in future situations.

- *Example*: "Every time I say the word 'calm,' I will instantly feel peaceful and relaxed."

6. Awakening from Self-Hypnosis

Once your suggestions are delivered, it's time to gently awaken from the hypnotic state. This is done gradually, with the intention of bringing the mind back to full awareness, while still feeling relaxed and positive.

Step-by-Step Awakening:

- *Reorient Yourself:* "Now, as I count from 1 to 5, I will gradually return to full awareness, bringing with me the calm and peace from this experience. One... slowly becoming more aware of your surroundings. Two... becoming more alert and awake. Three... feeling refreshed and relaxed. Four... almost fully awake. Five... eyes open, feeling calm, confident, and ready to move forward with your goal."

When you open your eyes, take a moment to reorient yourself, stretch, and notice the changes in how you feel.

7. Practicing Self-Hypnosis

To become proficient in self-hypnosis, practice regularly. The more you practice, the easier it becomes to enter a deep hypnotic state, and the more effective the process will be. Start with short sessions (10-15 minutes), and as you get more comfortable, you can extend the time and deepen the trance.

8. Common Challenges and Tips

- *Difficulty Relaxing:* If you find it difficult to relax, try listening to calming music or using a progressive relaxation recording to help guide you.
- *Mind Wandering*: If your mind wanders, gently bring your focus back to your breath, a mental image, or a specific suggestion. Don't judge yourself for it—just refocus.
- *Deepening the State*: If you don't feel deeply relaxed, use deepening techniques like counting down or visualizing a peaceful scene to help you go further into trance.

Self-hypnosis is a powerful tool for personal growth and achieving positive change. By following the steps of relaxation, deepening, and using positive suggestions, you can tap into your subconscious mind to overcome challenges, reduce stress, change habits, and improve your overall well-being. Regular practice can increase your ability to enter hypnosis quickly and effectively, empowering you to take control of your mental and emotional states.

Chapter 6: Deepening Hypnosis

Once you have successfully induced a hypnotic state, it's important to deepen that state to make the subject more receptive to suggestions and therapeutic interventions. Deepening techniques help to increase the subject's level of relaxation, focus, and receptivity by enhancing their hypnotic trance. In this chapter, we'll explore several methods to strengthen the trance state, including deepening scripts, countdowns, and other strategies that can lead to a more profound hypnotic experience.

1. Understanding the Importance of Deepening

Deepening hypnosis is crucial because the deeper the trance, the more effectively the subconscious mind becomes open to positive suggestions. While some individuals might experience a deep trance right away, others may require additional techniques to go further into the hypnotic state. Deepening increases the level of relaxation, reduces critical thinking, and enhances the subject's ability to make changes at a subconscious level.

Deepening techniques are especially useful in therapeutic settings, where a more profound level of trance may be required to facilitate healing, uncover memories, or alter behaviors.

1. Deepening Techniques

1. Counting Down

Counting down is one of the most widely used techniques to deepen hypnosis. It involves suggesting that the subject's relaxation will increase with each descending number, which helps to further relax the body and mind.

- *Step-by-Step:*
    - Begin by instructing the subject to focus on their breathing or the sensations in their body.
    - Suggest that with each number, they will feel more relaxed, and the deeper they go, the better they will feel.

Example Script:

- "I'm going to count backward from 10 to 1. With each number, you'll feel your body relaxing even more deeply. As the numbers decrease, your mind will quiet and drift deeper into this peaceful state."
- "Ten... feeling calm and peaceful. Nine... relaxing even deeper. Eight... your body is becoming heavier and more relaxed. Seven... feeling so at ease. Six... deeper still... with every breath you take, you go deeper into relaxation."
- Continue until reaching "one," suggesting that the subject is now in a deep, comfortable trance.

The countdown technique works by creating a rhythm and expectation of deeper relaxation with each number, giving the mind a simple, focused task that allows it to relax even more.

2. Visualizing Descending Stairs or an Elevator

Using imagery to deepen the trance is highly effective. By guiding the subject to imagine themselves descending stairs or riding an elevator down, you invoke a sense of deepening and relaxation as they mentally descend into a more profound state.

- *Step-by-Step:*
    - Invite the subject to visualize themselves standing at the top of a staircase or entering an elevator.
    - Suggest that as they move downward, they will feel more and more relaxed with every step or floor.

Example Script:

- "Now, imagine you are standing at the top of a beautiful staircase.

With each step you take, you go deeper and deeper into a state of relaxation. With each step, you feel more at peace, more comfortable. Step down... feeling more relaxed. Two steps down... sinking deeper into relaxation. Three steps down... letting go of all tension and stress."

- "You may also imagine yourself stepping into an elevator, pressing the button to descend. With each floor you pass, you go deeper into this calm, peaceful state of relaxation. As the elevator descends, you're going deeper and deeper into hypnosis."

This technique provides a mental focal point that guides the subject into deeper relaxation, using imagery to enhance the experience.

3. Fractionation (Inducing and Deepening Trance Cycles)
Fractionation is a technique that involves bringing the subject in and out of light trance states repeatedly. By doing so, you can enhance the depth of hypnosis because the subconscious mind becomes more accustomed to going deeper each time. This method can help the subject experience a heightened sense of relaxation and focus.

- *Step-by-Step:*
    - Begin by deepening the trance using any of the previous techniques.
    - After a period of deep relaxation, suggest that the subject will come back to full awareness, but only for a moment, and then return to an even deeper state of hypnosis.

Example Script:

- "I'm going to count from 1 to 3, and when I reach 3, you will come back to full awareness, feeling refreshed and alert. One... feeling more awake. Two... almost fully aware now. Three... wide awake. Take a deep breath in, and as you exhale, you'll go even deeper into relaxation, allowing yourself to sink into an even deeper, more peaceful state."

- Repeat this process several times, each time going deeper than the last.

The cycle of entering and exiting the trance state strengthens the subject's ability to go deeper with each repetition, and they begin to associate the state with a heightened sense of peace and receptivity.

4. Deepening Suggestions (Reinforcing Relaxation)
Deepening suggestions work by reinforcing the sense of relaxation and control over the physical and mental state. This can involve specific statements that increase the sense of heaviness, warmth, or peacefulness in the body.

- *Step-by-Step:*
    - Guide the subject to focus on their body sensations, asking them to relax specific parts of the body and deepen the relaxation with each breath.

Example Script:

- "As you continue to relax, you may notice a growing sense of warmth and heaviness spreading throughout your body. Your feet feel heavy and warm, as though they are sinking gently into the floor. With each breath, that feeling moves upward, and your legs, torso, and arms are becoming heavier and more relaxed. Your entire body is now calm, peaceful, and deeply at ease."
- "The deeper you relax, the more easily you can let go of any stress or tension. You feel safe and completely at ease in this state."

These types of suggestions deepen the hypnotic state by allowing the subject to fully engage with their body and deepen the sense of comfort and relaxation.

5. The "Sleep" Technique
The "sleep" technique involves suggesting that the subject will enter an even deeper trance by using the word "sleep," even though they remain fully conscious and aware. It is a psychological trigger that enhances the sense of relaxation and mental disconnection from the physical world.

- *Step-by-Step:*
  - After inducing a light trance, use the suggestion that the subject can go even deeper by hearing the word "sleep."
  - The subject is encouraged to relax further each time the word "sleep" is used.

Example Script:

- "Now, as I say the word 'sleep,' you'll allow yourself to drift even deeper into this wonderful state of relaxation. Sleep... deeper now... going deeper with each breath. Sleep... feel yourself sinking into a deeper state, where you feel completely relaxed and at peace."

This method reinforces the depth of the trance state through a simple suggestion, creating a powerful trigger that allows for deeper relaxation and focus.

6. Using Deepening Techniques in Combination

Often, the most effective way to deepen hypnosis is to combine several of the techniques above, as each has a unique benefit. For example, you can use counting down with deepening suggestions or combine visualization with fractionation for greater effect.

- *Example Combination:*
  - "Now, I will count backward from 10 to 1. With each number, your body will become more relaxed and heavy. As you relax more deeply, imagine yourself descending a beautiful staircase, going down to a deeper state with each step. Ten... stepping down, feeling calm. Nine... deeper still. Eight... the deeper you go, the more relaxed and at ease you feel."

By integrating multiple techniques, you can ensure that the subject reaches a profound state of hypnosis and remains there throughout the session.

Deepening techniques are essential for enhancing the effectiveness of hypnosis. By guiding the subject into a deeper trance, you increase their receptivity to suggestions, help them relax further, and open up their subconscious mind for therapeutic work. Whether you are counting down, using visualization, or reinforcing relaxation with deepening suggestions, the goal is always to guide the subject into a more profound, comfortable, and peaceful state. Mastering these techniques will ensure that you can help anyone enter a deep, receptive hypnotic state and achieve the desired results.

Signs of Deep Hypnosis

Recognizing when a person is in a deeply hypnotized state is essential for both the hypnotist and the subject. Being able to identify these signs allows the hypnotist to understand when the subject has entered a state where they are highly receptive to suggestions and can undergo therapeutic work. In this section, we'll explore the various physical, mental, and behavioral signs that indicate deep hypnosis.

1. Physical Signs of Deep Hypnosis

Hypnosis induces profound relaxation in the body, and many physical changes occur as a result. These changes are often subtle but can be observed with careful attention.

1.1. Muscle Relaxation and Heaviness

One of the first signs of deepening hypnosis is a noticeable relaxation of the muscles, often accompanied by a feeling of heaviness or limpness.

- *Heaviness*: The subject may report or appear to feel as though their body is becoming heavier. This often starts in the arms or legs and can spread to the entire body.
- *Limpness*: In a deep state, the subject's body may appear limp, with their posture softening and any tension releasing from the muscles.
- *Example*: The subject may have difficulty keeping their eyes open, their head may droop, or their arms may hang loosely at their sides. They may also be unable to consciously lift their limbs without effort.

1.2. Slow, Relaxed Breathing

As hypnosis deepens, the subject's breathing becomes slower, more rhythmic, and more relaxed.

- *Shallow or Deep Breathing*: Breathing may become slow, even, and shallow, indicating the relaxation of the diaphragm and chest muscles. In some cases, the subject may take deep, slow breaths as if entering a meditative state.
- *Example*: If you listen closely, the subject's breathing may become so slow and relaxed that it's almost imperceptible. You might notice the rise and fall of their chest or abdomen is very gradual and smooth.

1.3. Eye Changes

The eyes are one of the most telling indicators of hypnosis. As the subject enters deeper levels of trance, eye movements and the way the eyes appear can change significantly.

- *Eye Relaxation:* The eyes may become heavier, and the eyelids might flutter or begin to close involuntarily.
- *Glassy or Fixed Gaze*: In a deep state of hypnosis, the subject's eyes may appear "glassy," as though unfocused, or they may have a fixed, unfocused stare.
- *Lack of Blink Reflex*: Often, during deep hypnosis, the subject may stop blinking as frequently or at all. In some cases, their eyes may appear completely relaxed, and the eyelids may look heavy or droopy.
- *Example*: You may notice the subject's eyes are fixed on a point or have a blank, distant look. They may no longer exhibit a normal, conscious response to stimuli in the environment.

1.4. Relaxed Facial Muscles

In deep hypnosis, the facial muscles, particularly around the eyes, mouth, and forehead, relax significantly. This relaxation may lead to:

- *Softening of Facial Expressions*: The face becomes calm, with no tension or tightness around the forehead or jaw. A relaxed subject might appear more serene or at peace.

- *Drooping Eyelids:* The eyelids may droop or fully close, especially when the subject is in a deep trance, which is often accompanied by a deep state of relaxation.

2. Behavioral Signs of Deep Hypnosis

In addition to physical changes, there are several behavioral cues that indicate the subject has entered a deep trance. These can often be seen in the way they respond to commands or engage with the hypnotic process.

2.1. Unresponsiveness to External Stimuli

In deep hypnosis, the subject becomes less responsive to external distractions or stimuli. They may ignore sounds, movements, or anything that would normally grab their attention.

- *Reduced Awareness of Surroundings:* The subject's awareness of their environment diminishes, and they may become oblivious to sounds or people around them.
- *Focused Attention*: The subject will focus entirely on the hypnotic suggestions and may appear completely unaware of what's happening around them, as if in a trance-like state.
- *Example*: If there is background noise or conversation in the room, the subject might not react to it, even though they would normally respond. They are in a deep, internal state of focus.

2.2. Deeply Relaxed or Fixed Posture

In deep hypnosis, the subject may adopt a deeply relaxed posture or a fixed position. Their body may appear completely still, as they become less aware of their body's movements.

- *Frozen Posture*: In deep hypnosis, subjects may remain perfectly still, without shifting their body position, unless instructed otherwise.
- *Body Temperature Changes*: Some subjects may even experience a drop in body temperature, indicated by cold hands or feet.

- *Example*: You might notice the subject sitting or lying very still, almost as if frozen in time. If they are standing, they may sway gently or remain unmoving, like a statue.

2.3. Post-Hypnotic Suggestions and Responses
One of the clearest signs that a person is deeply hypnotized is their response to post-hypnotic suggestions, which can indicate a deeper level of receptivity.

- *Motor Response to Suggestions*: In some cases, subjects will exhibit motor responses that they are not consciously controlling. For example, their hand may rise without them thinking about it, or their eyes may blink automatically when instructed.
- *Increased Suggestibility:* A deep subject will often respond to suggestions much more readily and without hesitation.
- *Example*: If you suggest that their hand will rise when you count to three, they may unconsciously lift their hand without any physical effort or conscious awareness.

2.4. Changes in Speech Patterns
Speech can change when a subject enters a deep trance, often becoming slower, more rhythmic, or even more monotone.

- *Soft, Slow, or Slurred Speech:* In deep hypnosis, speech can slow down and become more deliberate. Some subjects may even speak in a more sluggish manner, as though their body and mind are deeply relaxed.
- *Altered Tone or Pitch*: The subject's voice might become softer or take on a different tone or pitch as they relax more deeply into the trance.
- *Example*: The subject may speak in a very calm, almost dream-like voice, and their responses may be slower or more drawn-out.

3. Psychological and Mental Signs of Deep Hypnosis

Mental changes are just as significant as physical ones and can indicate when someone has entered a deep hypnotic state.

3.1. Enhanced Focus and Absorption

Deep hypnosis typically leads to an enhanced state of focus, where the subject may become more absorbed in the hypnotic process.

- *Increased Concentration:* The person will likely show an increased focus on the hypnotist's voice or the suggested imagery, appearing to "zone out" from the external world.
- *Selective Attention*: They may seem to block out everything except the suggestions they are receiving, becoming highly focused on the hypnotist's voice or the task at hand.
- *Example*: The subject may appear deeply engrossed in the imagery or suggestions you're giving, almost as if they are not aware of their surroundings or anything that's not part of the hypnosis session.

3.2. Amnesia (Temporary Forgetfulness)
In deep hypnosis, the subject may experience temporary amnesia, meaning they forget certain parts of the session, including specific instructions or events.

- *Memory Gaps*: After awakening from the trance, the person may not remember everything that transpired during the hypnosis session, especially if they were in a very deep state.
- *Lack of Recall:* They may not recall the exact wording of suggestions or specific events from the session unless reminded.
- *Example*: After the session, the subject might not remember having their arm raised on command, or they might not recall certain details of their deep relaxation process.

Recognizing the signs of deep hypnosis allows the hypnotist to tailor the session to the subject's level of trance and adjust the pace or depth of the work being done. Physical signs like muscle relaxation, slowed breathing, and eye changes, as well as behavioral signs such as unresponsiveness and enhanced suggestibility, are all strong indicators that the subject is deeply hypnotized. By learning to identify these signs, you can more effectively guide the session and ensure that the subject remains in a state where positive change can occur.

Chapter 7: Hypnotic Suggestions

Hypnotic suggestions are one of the core components of hypnosis. They are the instructions or cues that a hypnotist provides to the subject while they are in a trance. Suggestions are what allow hypnosis to be therapeutic, as they can influence the subject's thoughts, behaviors, emotions, and physical sensations. This chapter will explore how suggestions work within hypnosis, the different types of suggestions, and how they can be applied effectively to create lasting change.

1. Understanding Hypnotic Suggestions

1.1. What Are Hypnotic Suggestions?

A hypnotic suggestion is a verbal or non-verbal cue given by the hypnotist while the subject is in a trance state, aimed at influencing the subject's thoughts, feelings, or behaviors. The power of suggestions lies in the subject's ability to focus intently on them while in a relaxed, highly suggestible state, making it easier for the subconscious mind to accept them.

Hypnotic suggestions are often used to address a variety of issues such as stress, anxiety, phobias, smoking cessation, pain management, and even performance enhancement. The key is that the subject is more open to suggestions in the hypnotic state, as their conscious mind is relaxed, and the subconscious is more receptive to change.

1.2. How Do Suggestions Work in Hypnosis?

The way suggestions work during hypnosis is rooted in the relationship between the conscious and subconscious mind. When a person is in hypnosis, the conscious mind relaxes, and the critical thinking processes are less active. This allows the subconscious mind to take center stage, where it is more malleable and open to accepting new ideas.

- *Conscious Mind:* In a normal, awake state, the conscious mind is constantly analyzing and questioning information. It filters out suggestions that seem unrealistic or untrue.
- *Subconscious Mind*: In the hypnotic state, the subconscious mind becomes more dominant. It accepts suggestions without the usual critical filtering and can then drive changes in thoughts, behaviors, and even bodily sensations.

Suggestions can range from simple instructions, like telling someone to relax, to more complex ones, like encouraging the person to change a particular habit or perception.

2. Types of Hypnotic Suggestions

There are several different types of suggestions that can be used in hypnosis. Each type serves a different purpose and can be tailored to suit the needs of the subject.

2.1. Direct Suggestions

Direct suggestions are straightforward instructions given to the subject while in a hypnotic state. These suggestions are clear, specific, and explicit. They are particularly effective when working with subjects who are highly suggestible and have a clear goal in mind.

- *Example*: "You will feel calm and relaxed in all situations from now on."
- *Usage*: Direct suggestions are often used for issues like stress reduction, pain management, and overcoming anxiety. They work best when the subject is receptive and open to change.
-

2.2. Indirect Suggestions

Indirect suggestions are more subtle and are often used when working with subjects who are less suggestible or resistant to direct commands. Indirect suggestions work by guiding the subject to a conclusion without explicitly telling them what to do. They often involve metaphor, stories, or suggestions that allow the subject to draw their own conclusions.

- *Example*: "Some people find that when they face stressful situations, they begin to feel a sense of calm, as if they have a deep inner strength that helps them manage the stress."
- *Usage*: Indirect suggestions are frequently used for people who are hesitant to change or those with more complex issues like deep-rooted fears or behavioral patterns.

2.3. Post-Hypnotic Suggestions

Post-hypnotic suggestions are instructions given during hypnosis that take effect after the subject has emerged from the trance. These suggestions trigger specific behaviors, thoughts, or emotions after the session has ended.

- *Example*: "From this moment on, whenever you feel the urge to smoke, you will take three deep breaths and feel a wave of relaxation sweep over you."
- *Usage*: Post-hypnotic suggestions are especially useful for breaking habits, such as smoking or overeating, as they create lasting changes that persist beyond the hypnosis session.

2.4. Conditional Suggestions

Conditional suggestions are statements that guide the subject to respond in a specific way if certain conditions are met. These suggestions are often linked to environmental cues or triggers that elicit a response once the subject encounters them.

- *Example*: "Every time you hear the sound of your phone ringing, you will feel calm and relaxed."
- *Usage*: Conditional suggestions are commonly used in habit change and behavioral therapy, as they create automatic responses to specific external stimuli.

2.5. Age Regression Suggestions

Age regression suggestions involve guiding the subject back to a previous time in their life, usually to a specific memory or event. This technique is used to help the subject access past experiences and emotions, which can often be therapeutic in addressing trauma, unresolved issues, or even phobias.

- *Example*: "I want you to imagine yourself as a young child, feeling safe and happy in that moment. What do you see around you? What do you hear?"
- *Usage*: Age regression can be used to uncover the root causes of phobias, trauma, or unwanted behaviors, helping the subject to reframe and heal old wounds.

3. Creating Effective Hypnotic Suggestions

Not all suggestions are equally effective. To ensure that suggestions work, they need to be crafted thoughtfully and be appropriate for the subject's goals. There are several key principles to keep in mind when creating effective hypnotic suggestions.

3.1. Clarity and Specificity

Suggestions should be clear, specific, and easy to understand. Vague or overly complex suggestions can confuse the subject and may not lead to the desired outcome.

- *Example*: Rather than saying, "You will feel better," say, "You will feel calm and relaxed, with a sense of peace and confidence in every situation."

3.2. Positive Language

Use positive language when phrasing suggestions. The subconscious mind responds more effectively to positive statements, as they create a sense of possibility and openness.

- *Example*: Instead of saying, "You won't feel anxious anymore," say, "You will feel calm and confident in all situations."

3.3. Present Tense

Suggestions should be phrased in the present tense, as though the change is already occurring. This creates a sense of immediacy and helps the subconscious mind to accept the suggestion as an ongoing reality.

- *Example*: "You are feeling more confident every day," rather than, "You will feel more confident in the future."

3.4. Personalization

Tailor the suggestions to the individual's specific needs, goals, and preferences. Personalized suggestions are more likely to resonate with the subject and lead to successful outcomes.

- *Example*: If a subject is trying to overcome a fear of public speaking, you might say, "Every time you speak in front of a group, you will feel calm and confident, enjoying the experience of sharing your thoughts."

4. The Power of Repetition

Repetition is key to reinforcing suggestions. The subconscious mind tends to accept suggestions more readily the more frequently they are repeated. When crafting your hypnotic suggestions, be sure to repeat them multiple times during the session, allowing the subject's subconscious mind to internalize them.

- *Example*: "You are confident and relaxed in all situations. You are confident and relaxed in all situations. You are confident and relaxed in all situations."

Repetition builds a stronger mental association with the suggestion and helps to make it a permanent part of the subject's thought patterns.

5. Testing and Adjusting Suggestions

It's important to test whether a suggestion is effective during the session and to adjust it if needed. Some subjects may respond immediately, while others might need additional reinforcement or a change in approach. Be attentive to the subject's responses, and if a suggestion isn't producing the desired effect, consider modifying it.

- *Example*: If a subject is not responding well to a relaxation suggestion, you might try adding more sensory detail to it, such as, "Imagine a wave of warmth flowing from your head to your toes, relaxing every muscle in your body."

Hypnotic suggestions are a powerful tool in hypnosis, allowing the hypnotist to influence the subject's thoughts, behaviors, and emotional state. By understanding how suggestions work and crafting them thoughtfully, you can help the subject achieve significant and lasting changes. Whether using direct, indirect, post-hypnotic, or conditional suggestions, the key is to ensure that they are clear, positive, personalized, and repeated. With practice, you will become skilled at using suggestions to facilitate profound transformation in your subjects.

Types of Hypnotic Suggestions

In hypnosis, suggestions are the primary method through which change is facilitated in the subconscious mind. There are various types of suggestions that can be used depending on the subject's needs, their level of suggestibility, and the desired outcome. The three main types of suggestions are **direct**, **indirect**, and **post-hypnotic** suggestions. Each of these has unique characteristics and uses. This section will break down these types and explain how and when they are most effective.

1. Direct Suggestions

What Are Direct Suggestions?

Direct suggestions are explicit and straightforward instructions or commands that are given to the subject during a hypnotic session. They are clear, simple, and unambiguous, making them effective when the subject is highly suggestible and ready for change. Direct suggestions work by speaking directly to the subject's subconscious mind, bypassing the critical conscious filters.

Characteristics of Direct Suggestions:

- *Clear and Specific:* They are simple, to the point, and often state exactly what is desired.
- *Authoritative Tone:* Direct suggestions often sound more like

commands, as they give the subject clear guidance on what to do or how to feel.

- *Effective with Highly Suggestible Subjects:* Direct suggestions tend to work best with subjects who are comfortable with hypnosis and are open to immediate change.

Examples of Direct Suggestions:

- "You will feel calm and relaxed whenever you take a deep breath."
- "From now on, you will have no cravings for cigarettes. You are a non-smoker."
- "You will feel more confident and at ease whenever you speak in public."

When to Use Direct Suggestions:
Direct suggestions are ideal when:

- The subject is receptive and willing to follow clear instructions.
- The goal is straightforward, such as managing stress, eliminating a simple phobia, or reinforcing positive behaviors.
- The subject has a high level of suggestibility and is not resistant to change.

2. Indirect Suggestions

What Are Indirect Suggestions?
Indirect suggestions are more subtle and less explicit than direct suggestions. Instead of commanding the subject to change, the hypnotist uses metaphor, storytelling, or vague language that guides the subconscious mind toward the desired outcome. Indirect suggestions are useful when the subject is less suggestible, more resistant, or when the goal requires a more flexible or nuanced approach.

Characteristics of Indirect Suggestions:

- *Subtle and Vague:* Indirect suggestions often involve implied meanings or metaphors, which allow the subject's subconscious mind to interpret the suggestion in a way that feels natural and non-threatening.

- *Engagement of the Imagination:* They often tap into the subject's imagination and personal experiences, making them feel more like self-discovery than direct command.
- *Non-Authoritative:* Rather than giving direct commands, indirect suggestions allow the subject to make their own connections to the desired outcome.

Examples of Indirect Suggestions:

- "Some people, when they begin to relax deeply, start to notice how calm and peaceful they feel."
- "Imagine a time when you felt completely at ease, and allow that feeling to grow stronger now."
- "You may begin to notice that, over time, certain things just seem to feel easier, almost effortlessly."

When to Use Indirect Suggestions:
Indirect suggestions are especially effective when:

- The subject is skeptical, resistant, or has trouble following direct commands.
- You are dealing with deeper issues, such as phobias, trauma, or negative beliefs.
- The subject is not fully aware of what the solution or change looks like, and you want to guide them toward discovering it themselves.
- The goal involves a gradual change or a shift in perception, rather than an immediate result.

3. Post-Hypnotic Suggestions
What Are Post-Hypnotic Suggestions?
Post-hypnotic suggestions are instructions given to the subject during hypnosis that are designed to take effect after the hypnotic session is over. These suggestions trigger specific behaviors, thoughts, or emotions once the subject is

back to their normal waking state. Post-hypnotic suggestions can have a lasting impact, as they can help reinforce new habits or changes long after the session has ended.

Characteristics of Post-Hypnotic Suggestions:

- *Time-Based*: These suggestions work after the hypnosis session, at a specific time or under specific conditions.
- *Behavioral Change*: They often prompt the subject to perform or feel something once they return to their daily life, such as breaking a bad habit, feeling calm in stressful situations, or achieving a new goal.
- *Triggerable by External Cues*: Post-hypnotic suggestions can be linked to external triggers, like a word, sound, or event that causes the subject to experience a desired behavior or feeling.

Examples of Post-Hypnotic Suggestions:

- "Whenever you hear a bell ring, you will feel a wave of calm and confidence wash over you."
- "From now on, whenever you feel the urge to eat unhealthy foods, you will find that you no longer desire them. Instead, you will naturally crave healthy options."
- "Every time you look at a specific object, you will feel a sense of motivation to complete your tasks with enthusiasm."

When to Use Post-Hypnotic Suggestions:
Post-hypnotic suggestions are ideal when:

- You want to create lasting, sustainable change that continues after the hypnosis session has ended.
- The goal is to break habits or reinforce positive behaviors that need to be triggered in real-life situations (e.g., stress management, smoking cessation, overcoming phobias).
- The subject requires long-term reinforcement of the changes made during the session.

<u>Comparison of the Three Types of Suggestions</u>

Type of Suggestion	Description	Best For	Example
Direct Suggestions	Clear and straightforward instructions.	Subjects who are highly suggestible or ready for change.	"You will feel relaxed and confident."
Indirect Suggestions	Subtle, vague, and often metaphorical instructions.	Subjects who are resistant, less suggestible, or when the goal requires flexibility.	"You may notice that the more you relax, the more confident you feel."
Post-Hypnotic Suggestions	Instructions that take effect after the session.	Creating lasting changes that persist after the hypnosis session.	"Every time you hear the word 'calm,' you will feel at ease."

4. Combining Suggestion Types

While each type of suggestion has its own benefits, they can also be combined to enhance the effectiveness of the session. For example, a hypnotist might use direct suggestions to initially guide the subject into a relaxed state, followed by indirect suggestions to deepen the experience and address underlying issues. Post-hypnotic suggestions can be added at the end of the session to reinforce lasting change in the subject's daily life.

- *Example Combination*: After guiding the subject into deep relaxation using direct suggestions like "Feel calm and relaxed now," the hypnotist might follow up with an indirect suggestion: "You may find that every time you take a deep breath, you feel more relaxed and peaceful," before adding a post-hypnotic suggestion: "From this moment on, whenever you take three deep breaths, you will automatically feel calm and relaxed, no matter the situation."

Each type of suggestion—direct, indirect, and post-hypnotic—plays an important role in the hypnosis process. Understanding how to use these suggestions effectively allows the hypnotist to tailor the experience to the subject's needs, whether they are looking for immediate relief, gradual change, or long-term results. By mastering these different suggestion techniques, you can enhance the effectiveness of your hypnosis sessions and create meaningful, lasting change for your subjects.

Crafting Effective Suggestions

Effective suggestions are at the heart of hypnosis and are essential for achieving desired outcomes. Crafting suggestions that are clear, precise, and effective is an art that involves understanding the mechanics of the subconscious mind and the principles of communication. This section will outline the key elements of creating powerful suggestions, including clarity, specificity, language, and the use of positive reinforcement.

1. The Importance of Clarity and Precision

Clarity in Hypnotic Suggestions

For a suggestion to be effective, it must be clear. The subconscious mind is sensitive to the way suggestions are phrased, and any ambiguity can reduce the suggestion's power. To ensure clarity:

- *Avoid Confusion:* Make sure that the suggestion is simple and straightforward, leaving no room for interpretation.
- *Use Simple Language:* Use everyday language that the subject can easily understand. Complex or technical terms can cause confusion and disrupt the flow of the session.
- *Be Direct*: Instead of saying, "You may feel more relaxed now," say, "You are now feeling calm and deeply relaxed."

Precision in Hypnotic Suggestions

Precise suggestions direct the subconscious mind to a specific outcome. Vague suggestions can cause the mind to wander or produce unpredictable results.

- *Be Specific:* Define exactly what you want the subject to experience or achieve. For example, instead of saying, "You will feel better," say, "You will feel calm, confident, and at ease every time you speak in public."
- *Visual and Sensory Detail:* Use sensory language (sight, sound, touch)

to create a vivid experience. For instance, "Imagine a warm, golden light surrounding you, making you feel peaceful and relaxed."

2. The Power of Positive Language

Hypnotic suggestions are far more effective when they are phrased positively, rather than negatively. The subconscious mind tends to focus on the language it hears, and negative suggestions can be misunderstood. Using positive, affirming language makes the suggestion easier to accept and reinforces the desired change.

Why Positive Language Matters

- *Focuses on What You Want, Not What You Don't Want:* The subconscious mind does not process negatives well. Telling someone "Don't feel anxious" might actually make them focus on anxiety, rather than its absence.
- *Encourages Empowerment:* Positive language motivates the subject and encourages confidence in their ability to achieve the desired result.

Examples of Positive Language

- *Negative*: "You will not feel anxious in these situations anymore."
- *Positive*: "You will feel calm and confident whenever you face challenges."
- *Negative*: "You won't be afraid of public speaking."
- *Positive*: "You will feel confident, relaxed, and at ease when speaking in front of others."

3. Using the Present Tense

The subconscious mind responds more readily to suggestions that are phrased in the present tense, as if the change is already happening or has already occurred. By using the present tense, the suggestion feels immediate and real, encouraging the subject's mind to accept it as part of their current reality.

Why the Present Tense is Effective

- *Creates a Sense of Immediacy*: It convinces the subconscious mind that the desired change is already happening.
- *Reinforces Current Behavior or Feelings:* The present tense suggestion encourages the subject to believe that the change is occurring now, rather than at some point in the future.

Examples of Present Tense Suggestions

- "You feel calm and relaxed right now, and this feeling will continue throughout your day."
- "You are confident and focused, and this confidence grows stronger with each passing day."

4. Tailoring Suggestions to the Individual

Effective suggestions should be personalized to the subject's needs, desires, and life experiences. A one-size-fits-all approach is rarely as effective as one that speaks to the subject's unique goals or challenges.

Personalization of Suggestions

- *Use Their Own Language:* Incorporate words or phrases that the subject naturally uses or identifies with. This makes the suggestion feel more relatable and genuine.
- *Address Specific Goals:* Customize the suggestions to focus on what the subject wants to achieve. If they are working on reducing stress, suggest relaxation and calm. If they are working on a behavior change, tailor the suggestion to that particular change.

Example of Tailored Suggestions

- *For Someone Working on Stress:* "Each time you encounter stress, you will automatically breathe deeply, and you will feel a wave of relaxation wash over you."
- *For Someone Overcoming Fear of Public Speaking*: "When you stand in front of a group, you will feel calm, confident, and fully in control. You will speak clearly, without fear, and enjoy the experience."

5. Using Sensory Language

One of the most powerful tools in crafting effective suggestions is using sensory language. The subconscious mind processes sensory input as if it were real, so the more vivid and detailed the sensory description, the more effective the suggestion will be.

Sensory Language and Its Impact

- *Engages the Subconscious Mind:* The more the suggestion involves the senses, the easier it is for the subconscious mind to accept it as an experience.
- *Creates Vivid Mental Images:* Sensory-rich suggestions help the subject vividly imagine the desired change, making it feel more real and achievable.

Examples of Sensory Language

- "Imagine feeling a warm, soothing sensation spreading through your body, starting from your feet and moving up to your head."
- "Picture yourself walking into a room with a bright, welcoming light. You feel a sense of calm as you inhale the fresh, clean air around you."

6. Using Repetition and Reinforcement

Repetition is one of the most effective techniques in hypnosis. The more a suggestion is repeated, the more deeply it penetrates the subconscious mind. Repeating suggestions during the session allows the mind to absorb the message and make it a part of the subject's habitual thinking.

Repetition Techniques

- *Repeat Key Phrases:* Using the same suggestion multiple times helps to cement it in the subconscious.
- *Reinforce Positive Change:* Repeating the suggestion at different points in the session ensures that the subconscious mind hears it frequently, which builds trust in the new behavior or thought pattern.

- *Vary the Phrasing:* You can repeat the suggestion in different forms to increase its effectiveness. For example: "You are feeling confident" can be repeated as "With every passing moment, your confidence grows."

Example of Repetition in Suggestions

- "You feel more and more relaxed with every breath you take. You are relaxing deeper and deeper with each breath. Every breath you take brings you deeper into relaxation."

7. Timing and Pacing

The way suggestions are delivered can impact their effectiveness. It's important to pace the suggestions and timing, so the subject can process and absorb them properly.

Effective Pacing of Suggestions

- *Allow Time for Absorption:* Don't rush through suggestions. Give the subject time to experience and absorb each one.
- *Pace with the Subject's Breathing:* Often, it's effective to synchronize suggestions with the subject's breathing patterns. This helps reinforce the suggestion's calming or energizing effect.

Example of Pacing

- "As you breathe in, you feel calmness entering your body... and as you breathe out, you release any tension or stress."

8. Using Future-Oriented Suggestions

Future-oriented suggestions focus on how the subject will feel or behave after the session is over. These suggestions help the subject visualize themselves successfully implementing the changes in real-life situations.

Why Future-Oriented Suggestions Work

- *Helps Build Confidence:* They allow the subject to see themselves succeeding, which increases their belief that they can follow through

on the changes.
- *Aligns with Goals:* Future-oriented suggestions help reinforce the goal and create a mental map for success.

Examples of Future-Oriented Suggestions

- "In the days to come, you will feel more and more confident in every situation."
- "As you go about your day, you will notice that you automatically feel relaxed and at ease."

Crafting effective suggestions is an essential skill for any hypnotist. Clear, precise, and well-structured suggestions that use positive language, sensory-rich detail, and are tailored to the individual can significantly enhance the success of the hypnosis session. By mastering these principles—clarity, positive framing, specificity, sensory engagement, and repetition—you can create powerful suggestions that lead to lasting changes in your subject's behavior, thoughts, and emotions.

Working with Resistance: How to Deal with Subjects Who Resist Suggestions

Resistance is a common challenge in hypnosis, and it can occur for many reasons. Whether due to skepticism, fear, lack of trust, or subconscious defense mechanisms, resistance can prevent effective change. However, with the right approach, resistance can be managed and even overcome. This section outlines strategies for handling resistant subjects and ensuring that hypnosis sessions are productive and successful.

1. Understanding Resistance

What is Resistance?

Resistance in hypnosis refers to the subject's reluctance, reluctance to follow suggestions, or an active block that prevents the desired changes from occurring. It can manifest in different ways, such as:

- *Physical Discomfort:* Fidgeting, muscle tension, or nervous habits.
- *Mental Resistance:* Doubt, skepticism, or inner conflict.
- *Emotional Resistance*: Feelings of fear, anxiety, or reluctance to change.

Common Causes of Resistance:

- *Fear of Losing Control:* Some individuals worry that they will lose control during hypnosis and be forced to do things against their will.
- *Skepticism*: Many subjects doubt the effectiveness of hypnosis or may not fully believe in its power.
- *Past Experiences*: Negative past experiences with hypnosis or therapy may lead to reluctance or fear.
- *Subconscious Protection*: The subconscious mind may resist suggestions if it perceives the change as threatening or conflicting with the individual's current self-image or beliefs.

By understanding the underlying causes of resistance, you can choose the best strategies to help the subject move past it.

2. Building Trust and Rapport

Before attempting to address resistance, it's crucial to have a strong foundation of trust and rapport with the subject. If they don't feel safe or comfortable, resistance is likely to increase.

How to Build Trust:

- *Be Patient and Compassionate:* Acknowledge the subject's concerns without judgment. Create a supportive environment where they feel comfortable expressing their fears or doubts.
- *Clarify the Process*: Explain the hypnosis process clearly so that the subject understands what will happen. This can help reduce fear and skepticism.
- *Use Reassurance*: Remind the subject that they are in control at all times. Hypnosis is a cooperative process, and they cannot be made to

do anything against their will.

- *Respect Boundaries*: If the subject is uncomfortable with a particular suggestion or technique, respect their boundaries and adjust accordingly.

1. Identifying and Addressing Specific Forms of Resistance
2.

1. Skepticism
Many people are skeptical about hypnosis, often due to misconceptions or lack of understanding. Skepticism can make it difficult for a subject to fully relax and enter a receptive state.

How to Handle Skepticism:

- *Provide Clear Explanations:* Explain the process of hypnosis in simple terms. Clarify that it is a natural, focused state of awareness, not "mind control."
- *Use a Calm and Reassuring Voice:* Maintain a calm, confident tone to build trust. This will help the subject relax and feel more open to the process.
- *Use a Short Test Induction*: Sometimes, starting with a short, simple induction (like an arm levitation or light relaxation technique) can demonstrate that hypnosis works, which can dissolve skepticism.

2. Fear of Losing Control
A subject's fear of losing control during hypnosis can be a major source of resistance. They may worry that they will say or do something they don't want to do.

How to Handle Fear of Losing Control:

- *Emphasize Control:* Reassure the subject that they are always in control during the session and that they cannot be made to do anything they do not want to do.
- *Introduce Relaxation and Comforting Techniques*: Before starting any

deeper work, ensure the subject is fully relaxed and calm. Utilize progressive relaxation or other calming techniques to reduce anxiety and build confidence.

- *Use Positive Reinforcement:* Reinforce that they are doing well and in control throughout the session, praising their willingness to participate.

3. Subconscious Blocks

Sometimes, resistance comes from the subconscious mind, which may perceive the change as threatening or unnecessary. This could be linked to deeply held beliefs or fears that the subject may not even be consciously aware of.

How to Handle Subconscious Blocks:

- *Use Gentle and Indirect Suggestions:* When the subconscious resists direct suggestions, try using indirect language, metaphors, or storytelling that helps the mind accept change more naturally.
- *Work with the Resistance*: Instead of fighting the resistance, use it to your advantage. For example, you might suggest that "any resistance you may feel is simply a sign of how much the mind wants to protect you, and it's okay to let go of that protection now."
- *Gradual Approach*: If the subject is resistant to making a big change, try taking small steps. Gradually increase the intensity of the suggestions as the subject becomes more comfortable.

4. Physical Resistance (Tension, Fidgeting)

Physical resistance can manifest as fidgeting, muscle tension, or difficulty staying still. This can signal a lack of relaxation, which may hinder the success of hypnosis.

How to Handle Physical Resistance:

- *Check Comfort Levels:* Ensure the subject is comfortable in their position. Physical discomfort can be a source of resistance.
- *Progressive Relaxation*: Use relaxation techniques like progressive muscle relaxation to ease physical tension and help the subject get

into a deeper state of relaxation.

- *Guide Breathwork*: Focus on deep, slow breathing to help the subject relax. Encourage them to breathe deeply and slowly to release physical tension.

1. *Techniques for Overcoming Resistance*
2.

1. Reframing

Reframing involves changing the way a subject views a particular situation or feeling. It helps the subject understand their resistance in a new light, making it easier to overcome.

How to Use Reframing:

- *Acknowledge the Resistance:* Start by acknowledging the resistance in a non-judgmental way. For example, "It's completely normal to feel some resistance when trying something new."
- *Introduce a Positive Perspective*: Then, offer a positive perspective, such as "Resistance is simply the mind's way of protecting you, but you are safe, and it is okay to let go of that protection now."
- *Offer the Subject Control:* Reinforce that they have control over the process, and they can choose to release their resistance when they are ready.

2. Fractionation

Fractionation is a technique in which the hypnotist brings the subject in and out of hypnosis multiple times. This can help desensitize the subject to resistance and create stronger, more lasting change.

How to Use Fractionation:

- *Induce a Light Trance*: Start by bringing the subject into a light trance.
- *Awaken the Subject:* Gently bring the subject out of hypnosis for a brief moment, then re-induce the trance.

- *Repeat the Process:* By repeatedly bringing the subject in and out of the hypnotic state, you can help them overcome resistance and strengthen their ability to enter hypnosis.

3. Direct and Indirect Approaches

A combination of direct and indirect suggestions can be effective in breaking resistance. For example, while using direct suggestions to guide the subject toward relaxation, you can incorporate indirect suggestions that bypass the conscious resistance.

How to Use Direct and Indirect Suggestions Together:

- *Direct Suggestions:* "You are now feeling more relaxed with each breath you take."
- *Indirect Suggestions:* "As you breathe in deeply, you may notice that the deeper you relax, the more confident and at ease you feel."

Resistance is a natural part of the hypnotic process and can arise for a variety of reasons, but it can be managed effectively with patience, empathy, and the right techniques. Building trust, understanding the root cause of resistance, and using methods like reframing, fractionation, and direct/indirect suggestions are key strategies for overcoming resistance. By maintaining a calm and supportive approach, you can guide even the most resistant subjects toward successful outcomes.

Chapter 8: Applications of Hypnosis

Hypnosis is a powerful tool that has been used for centuries in various fields, particularly in therapeutic settings. Its ability to access the subconscious mind allows for profound changes in behavior, emotional responses, and even physical sensations. This chapter will explore the key therapeutic uses of hypnosis, including pain management, stress relief, habit change, and addressing psychological issues.

1. Therapeutic Uses of Hypnosis

Hypnosis is widely recognized for its therapeutic potential in treating a variety of conditions. It is a non-invasive, holistic approach that can complement or enhance traditional medical treatments. Below are the primary therapeutic uses of hypnosis:

Pain Management

One of the most well-known and researched applications of hypnosis is in pain management. Hypnosis can help reduce pain perception, increase pain tolerance, and promote healing in individuals experiencing acute or chronic pain.

How Hypnosis Helps with Pain:

- *Pain Reduction*: Hypnosis can alter the way the brain processes pain signals, reducing the sensation of pain. Through focused relaxation and guided imagery, the subject's attention is directed away from pain, reducing its intensity.
- *Increased Pain Tolerance*: Hypnosis can help individuals build a higher tolerance for pain, especially during medical procedures or rehabilitation.
- *Enhancing Healing*: By promoting relaxation and reducing stress,

hypnosis can accelerate the body's natural healing process.

- *Chronic Pain Conditions:* Hypnosis has been used to treat conditions like fibromyalgia, arthritis, back pain, and migraines by reducing the emotional and physical components of pain.

Example of a Pain Management Technique:

- A typical hypnosis session for pain management may involve guiding the subject into a deeply relaxed state, then using visualizations such as imagining the pain as a color or shape that can be "melted away" or "shifted" to a less intense sensation.

Stress Relief and Anxiety Reduction

Stress and anxiety are among the most common reasons people seek therapeutic hypnosis. Hypnosis works by accessing the subconscious mind to help the subject reframe stressful thoughts and reduce the body's physiological stress responses.

How Hypnosis Helps with Stress and Anxiety:

- *Relaxation Response*: Through deep relaxation, hypnosis triggers the body's natural "relaxation response," reducing heart rate, lowering blood pressure, and easing muscle tension.
- *Reducing Negative Thought Patterns*: Hypnosis can help shift negative thinking and stress-inducing thought patterns by reframing beliefs and enhancing positive, calming thoughts.
- *Managing Anxiety*: In individuals with anxiety disorders, hypnosis can be used to reduce feelings of panic, worry, and fear by teaching the mind to respond differently to triggers.
- *Decreasing Cortisol:* Chronic stress leads to elevated cortisol levels, which are linked to various health issues. Hypnosis helps reduce cortisol levels, fostering a sense of calm and well-being.

Example of a Stress Relief Technique:

- A common method for stress relief in hypnosis involves progressive relaxation, where the hypnotist guides the subject through each part of the body, releasing tension and promoting deep calm. This is often followed by suggestions of peace and tranquility.

Habit Change (Smoking, Weight Loss, Nail Biting, etc.)
Hypnosis is widely used in helping individuals break negative habits, whether it's smoking, overeating, nail-biting, or procrastination. The power of hypnosis lies in its ability to access the subconscious mind, where many of these habits are deeply ingrained.

How Hypnosis Helps with Habit Change:

- *Reprogramming the Subconscious*: Habits are often formed through repetitive thoughts and behaviors that become automatic. Hypnosis can help reprogram the subconscious mind to break these patterns and replace them with healthier choices.
- *Behavior Modification*: Through suggestions, hypnosis helps individuals change their thought processes and behaviors, making it easier for them to adopt new, positive habits.
- *Enhancing Willpower and Motivation*: Hypnosis strengthens an individual's commitment to making positive changes by boosting self-control, motivation, and determination.

Examples of Habit Change Techniques:

- *Smoking Cessation*: Hypnosis for smoking cessation typically involves suggestions that help the subject envision themselves as a non-smoker and associate smoking with negative sensations, like unpleasant taste or smell.
- *Weight Loss:* In hypnosis for weight loss, the subject may be guided to make healthier food choices, exercise more, and see themselves as reaching their ideal weight. Additionally, the hypnotist might use techniques like "gastric band" hypnosis, where the subject visualizes their stomach shrinking, reducing their appetite.

2. Hypnosis for Psychological Issues

Hypnosis is also widely used to address various psychological issues, particularly those that are deeply rooted in the subconscious mind. These include conditions such as anxiety, depression, phobias, PTSD, and more.

Anxiety and Panic Disorders

Hypnosis can be particularly effective in managing anxiety and panic disorders. The therapeutic techniques used in hypnosis can help individuals control their anxious thoughts and physical reactions, which are often exacerbated by negative thinking patterns.

How Hypnosis Helps with Anxiety and Panic:

- *Relaxation and Grounding*: Hypnosis can induce a deeply relaxed state, reducing the physical symptoms of anxiety such as rapid heartbeat and shallow breathing.
- *Changing Thought Patterns*: Through suggestions and reframing, hypnosis can alter the subconscious thought patterns that contribute to anxiety, helping individuals feel more in control.
- *Building Resilience*: Hypnosis helps build emotional resilience by teaching the subject to remain calm and composed when faced with anxiety-inducing situations.

Example of an Anxiety Technique:

- A common hypnosis technique for anxiety involves visualizing a "safe place," where the subject can retreat mentally whenever they feel stressed or anxious. The therapist then uses calming suggestions to reinforce a sense of safety and relaxation.

Phobias and Fears

Hypnosis is often used to treat phobias, such as fear of flying, spiders, heights, or social situations. The therapeutic goal is to alter the subconscious associations that trigger irrational fear and replace them with more neutral or positive associations.

How Hypnosis Helps with Phobias:

- *Desensitization*: Through gradual exposure or mental imagery, hypnosis can help desensitize the subject to the feared object or situation. This technique reduces the intensity of the emotional response.
- *Reframing the Fear*: By helping the subject reframe their perceptions of the fear, hypnosis enables them to respond with calmness and control rather than panic.
- *Anchoring Positive Feelings*: Hypnosis can anchor feelings of calmness and confidence to situations that previously triggered fear, so that the subject can remain relaxed in future encounters.

Example of Phobia Treatment:

- For a person with a fear of flying, the hypnotist may guide the subject through a relaxation process and then use imagery to help them imagine a peaceful flight experience. Over time, the subject will associate flying with feelings of calm and relaxation.

Post-Traumatic Stress Disorder (PTSD)

Hypnosis is increasingly used to treat PTSD by helping individuals confront traumatic memories in a safe and controlled manner. It allows the subconscious mind to process unresolved emotions and experiences, reducing their emotional impact.

How Hypnosis Helps with PTSD:

- *Reprocessing Traumatic Memories:* Under hypnosis, the subject may revisit traumatic memories in a controlled and safe environment, allowing them to process and release negative emotions.
- *Reframing Traumatic Events*: Hypnosis can help the individual reinterpret the traumatic event, reducing its emotional charge and integrating it into their life story in a way that is less distressing.
- *Stress Relief:* Hypnosis can also help reduce the physical and emotional tension associated with PTSD, offering relaxation and relief from the hyperarousal symptoms that often accompany the

disorder.

Example of PTSD Treatment:

- A therapist may use a technique known as "regression" to help the subject revisit a traumatic event in a safe manner. The therapist will guide the subject to view the event from a detached perspective, using positive suggestions to help them release feelings of fear or helplessness.

Hypnosis offers a wide range of therapeutic applications that can help individuals overcome physical, emotional, and psychological challenges. Whether it's managing pain, reducing stress, overcoming bad habits, or addressing psychological issues, hypnosis provides a non-invasive, effective solution that taps into the power of the subconscious mind. By utilizing these therapeutic techniques, individuals can experience lasting transformation and improved well-being.

Performance and Confidence Enhancement: Using Hypnosis for Self-Improvement and Achieving Goals

Hypnosis is a powerful tool not only for addressing psychological and physical issues but also for enhancing performance and boosting confidence. Whether for athletes aiming to improve their skills, professionals seeking success in their careers, or individuals working to achieve personal goals, hypnosis can be a catalyst for personal growth and achievement. By accessing the subconscious mind, hypnosis can help individuals overcome self-limiting beliefs, increase motivation, and enhance focus, allowing them to reach their full potential.

1. How Hypnosis Enhances Performance

Performance enhancement through hypnosis is based on the principle that the subconscious mind can influence conscious behaviors, habits, and skills. By using hypnosis, individuals can improve their performance in a variety of fields, including sports, public speaking, work, or any activity that requires focus, skill, or emotional regulation.

How Hypnosis Enhances Performance:

- *Improving Focus and Concentration:* Hypnosis helps individuals focus their attention on specific tasks by quieting mental distractions and enhancing concentration. This allows them to remain fully engaged in their performance without being sidetracked by extraneous thoughts.
- *Overcoming Mental Blocks:* Whether it's a performance anxiety or a mental block that prevents individuals from reaching their potential, hypnosis can help break through these barriers by altering subconscious beliefs and fears that limit their abilities.
- *Building Mental Resilience*: Hypnosis can increase mental resilience by teaching individuals how to stay calm and composed under pressure. This is particularly beneficial in high-stress situations such as competitions, presentations, or exams.
- *Visualization and Mental Rehearsal*: Through guided imagery and visualization, hypnosis allows individuals to mentally rehearse their performance, improving their skill level and confidence. This process prepares the brain for real-life execution, reinforcing positive outcomes.

Example of Performance Enhancement Technique:

- An athlete preparing for a competition may use hypnosis to visualize a perfect performance. The therapist guides them through a detailed mental rehearsal, where the athlete sees themselves performing flawlessly, feeling confident and in control throughout the event.

2. Using Hypnosis for Confidence Building

Confidence is a critical factor in achieving success, yet many individuals struggle with self-doubt, fear of failure, or insecurity. Hypnosis can help individuals build unshakable confidence by transforming limiting beliefs, promoting self-acceptance, and strengthening their sense of self-worth.

How Hypnosis Boosts Confidence:

- *Changing Negative Self-Talk:* Hypnosis can help replace negative thoughts with positive affirmations and empowering beliefs. By altering the subconscious patterns of self-criticism, individuals can develop a more optimistic outlook and greater self-belief.
- *Strengthening Self-Worth:* Hypnosis works to foster self-love and self-acceptance, allowing individuals to view themselves in a more positive light. It encourages individuals to recognize their strengths, talents, and potential.
- *Breaking Free from Fear of Failure:* Fear of failure often stems from past experiences or limiting beliefs. Hypnosis can help reframe these fears, encouraging individuals to embrace challenges as opportunities for growth rather than threats.
- *Improving Body Language:* Confidence is often reflected in body language. Hypnosis can influence subconscious behaviors, encouraging the individual to stand taller, make eye contact, and express themselves assertively.

Example of Confidence Enhancement Technique:

- In a hypnosis session focused on building confidence, the subject may be guided through a process where they imagine themselves in different scenarios (e.g., a meeting, a public speech, or a social event). The therapist reinforces the belief that they are calm, assertive, and confident in each of these situations, planting the idea that they can naturally perform with self-assurance.

3. Goal Achievement and Motivation

Hypnosis can be incredibly effective for goal setting and achievement by aligning the subconscious mind with conscious desires. Often, individuals set goals but struggle with follow-through due to lack of motivation, procrastination, or internal resistance. Hypnosis helps to enhance motivation by embedding powerful affirmations and desires in the subconscious mind, ensuring that goals are pursued with energy and determination.

How Hypnosis Aids in Goal Achievement:

- *Clarifying Goals:* Hypnosis can help individuals gain clarity on their goals by guiding them through the process of defining what they truly want. This may involve visualizing the desired outcome and recognizing the steps needed to reach it.
- *Increasing Motivation:* Hypnosis can embed positive suggestions related to motivation, helping individuals feel inspired to take consistent action toward their goals. By visualizing the rewards and satisfaction of achieving their goals, motivation is naturally enhanced.
- *Overcoming Procrastination:* Procrastination often arises from subconscious fears or limiting beliefs. Hypnosis helps identify the root cause of procrastination and replaces it with positive beliefs about taking action and completing tasks on time.
- *Building Persistence and Discipline:* Hypnosis can instill a sense of persistence and commitment, which is key for achieving long-term goals. By reinforcing the idea of steady progress and discipline, individuals become more dedicated to their success.

Example of Goal Achievement Technique:

- An individual seeking career advancement might use hypnosis to visualize themselves succeeding in their job, receiving promotions, and achieving their career goals. Throughout the session, the hypnotist may reinforce the idea that they are fully capable, hardworking, and focused on their professional aspirations.

4. Overcoming Performance Anxiety

Performance anxiety is a common challenge that affects individuals in many areas, including public speaking, sports, and work presentations. The fear of failure, judgment, or inadequacy can hinder performance and reduce overall confidence. Hypnosis can help individuals confront these anxieties, reframe their fears, and perform at their best.

How Hypnosis Helps with Performance Anxiety:

- *Reducing Fear of Judgment:* Hypnosis can help individuals let go of the fear of being judged or criticized by others. By shifting their focus to the task at hand and reframing negative perceptions, they can become more confident in their abilities.

- *Relaxation and Calmness:* Hypnosis induces deep relaxation, which can help individuals remain calm and composed during high-pressure situations. It helps lower physical symptoms of anxiety such as rapid heartbeat, shallow breathing, and sweating.
- *Positive Visualization*: Hypnosis can guide the individual through positive mental rehearsals, where they visualize themselves succeeding in their performance. By repeatedly imagining success, the individual develops a sense of mastery and reduces anxiety.
- *Creating a "Confidence Anchor":* Hypnosis can help individuals create a physical or mental "anchor" (a gesture, a phrase, or an image) that they can use to trigger feelings of confidence and calmness whenever they are about to perform.

Example of Overcoming Performance Anxiety Technique:

- A public speaker suffering from stage fright might be guided through hypnosis to imagine themselves walking onto the stage, feeling calm, confident, and composed. The therapist might also suggest that whenever they feel nervous before a presentation, they can take a deep breath and trigger their "confidence anchor," instantly calming their nerves.

5. Hypnosis for Creativity and Problem-Solving

In addition to enhancing confidence and performance, hypnosis can also unlock creativity and improve problem-solving abilities. Many individuals experience mental blocks that prevent them from thinking clearly or tapping into their creative potential. Hypnosis can help open the subconscious mind to new ideas, perspectives, and solutions.

How Hypnosis Enhances Creativity:

- *Accessing the Subconscious Mind:* Hypnosis allows individuals to access deeper levels of consciousness, where creative ideas and solutions may reside. By bypassing the critical conscious mind, the subject can tap into the intuitive and creative aspects of the subconscious.

- *Breaking Mental Blocks*: Hypnosis helps individuals identify and break through creative blocks, such as fear of failure or perfectionism, allowing the free flow of ideas and innovation.
- *Encouraging Divergent Thinking:* Hypnosis can enhance divergent thinking, which is the ability to generate a wide variety of ideas or solutions. This is particularly useful in creative fields such as writing, art, or problem-solving in business or technology.

Example of Creativity Enhancement Technique:

- A writer experiencing writer's block might use hypnosis to enter a relaxed state, then visualize themselves writing effortlessly, with ideas flowing freely. They may be guided to access their creative subconscious, where new story ideas or plot twists are waiting to be discovered.

Hypnosis is a versatile tool for enhancing performance and confidence. It can help individuals improve their focus, overcome mental barriers, boost self-belief, and achieve their goals. By working with the subconscious mind, hypnosis enables individuals to break free from limiting beliefs, build resilience, and tap into their true potential. Whether it's for enhancing athletic performance, excelling in a career, or simply improving self-confidence, hypnosis provides a powerful, transformative tool for personal development.

Hypnosis for Habit Change: Techniques for Overcoming Bad Habits

Hypnosis is a powerful tool for breaking unwanted habits and adopting healthier behaviors. Whether someone is struggling with smoking, overeating, nail-biting, or procrastination, hypnosis can help address the root causes of these habits and replace them with more positive, empowering behaviors. By working with the subconscious mind, hypnosis can facilitate deep behavioral changes, making it easier to break free from the patterns that hold individuals back.

1. How Hypnosis Helps with Habit Change

Habits, whether they are positive or negative, are largely stored in the subconscious mind. This is where repeated behaviors and automatic responses are formed. Hypnosis works by bypassing the conscious mind and communicating directly with the subconscious, which is where habits are entrenched. With the power of suggestion, hypnosis can reprogram the subconscious mind, breaking the cycle of undesirable behaviors and replacing them with healthier, more productive actions.

How Hypnosis Facilitates Habit Change:

- *Accessing the Subconscious Mind*: Many habits are the result of subconscious programming. Hypnosis allows individuals to access this deeper part of the mind, where they can identify the triggers and emotional connections tied to the habit.
- *Reframing the Habit:* Hypnosis helps reframe the way individuals perceive their habits. For example, someone trying to quit smoking may begin to associate smoking with unpleasant sensations, while associating healthy alternatives with positive feelings.
- *Creating New Behavioral Patterns:* Through repeated suggestions and visualization, hypnosis encourages new, positive behavioral patterns, gradually replacing the old habit with a healthier one.
- *Boosting Motivation and Willpower:* Hypnosis can increase an individual's motivation to succeed by strengthening their internal drive, reinforcing their commitment to breaking the habit and achieving their desired behavior.

2. Smoking Cessation through Hypnosis

Smoking is one of the most common habits that people seek to change through hypnosis. Cigarette smoking is not only a physical addiction but also a deeply ingrained habit tied to emotional and psychological triggers. Hypnosis works to address both the physical craving and the psychological attachment to smoking.

How Hypnosis Helps with Smoking Cessation:

- *Breaking the Psychological Association: Hypnosis* can help break the psychological triggers associated with smoking, such as the habit of reaching for a cigarette when stressed or after meals. By addressing these triggers in the subconscious, individuals can find new, healthier ways to cope.
- *Reprogramming the Mind*: Through suggestion, hypnosis can reframe the desire to smoke. For example, the individual might be encouraged to visualize cigarettes as unpleasant or disgusting, thereby reducing the appeal of smoking.
- *Strengthening the Desire to Quit:* Hypnosis can reinforce the individual's desire to quit smoking, helping them feel confident in their ability to quit for good. It can also enhance willpower and determination, especially during moments of temptation.
- *Reducing Withdrawal Symptoms:* While nicotine addiction is a physical factor in smoking, hypnosis can also help alleviate withdrawal symptoms by boosting relaxation, reducing cravings, and providing positive reinforcement.
-

Example of Smoking Cessation Technique:

- A smoking cessation hypnosis session might involve guiding the individual into a relaxed state, then using suggestions that associate smoking with feelings of disgust, while simultaneously reinforcing positive behaviors such as taking deep breaths or drinking water when the urge to smoke arises. Additionally, visualizations of a healthier, smoke-free lifestyle can be used to motivate and empower the individual.

3. Overcoming Overeating and Weight Loss

Overeating is another common habit that hypnosis is highly effective at addressing. Often, overeating is driven by emotional triggers, stress, or learned behaviors that cause individuals to consume more food than they need. Hypnosis helps individuals identify the root causes of their overeating and retrains their subconscious mind to respond to food in a healthier way.

How Hypnosis Helps with Overeating:

- *Addressing Emotional Eating:* Hypnosis can help individuals recognize when they are eating due to emotions like stress, boredom, or anxiety, rather than hunger. By teaching new coping strategies for managing emotions, hypnosis helps individuals break the cycle of emotional eating.
- *Creating Healthy Associations with Food:* Hypnosis can reframe the way individuals view food. For example, they might associate healthy foods with positive feelings, and unhealthy foods with negative feelings. This shift helps them make healthier choices more naturally.
- *Boosting Motivation for Exercise:* Hypnosis can increase an individual's motivation to exercise, which often plays a key role in weight loss and maintaining a healthy lifestyle. It can reinforce the benefits of regular physical activity and help individuals feel more energized and eager to move their bodies.
- *Promoting Portion Control:* Hypnosis can encourage mindful eating and portion control by suggesting that the individual feels full after smaller portions of food. This can help them avoid overeating and develop healthier eating habits.

Example of Overeating and Weight Loss Technique:

- A hypnosis session focused on overeating may involve guiding the individual to visualize themselves eating healthy, satisfying meals in moderate portions. The hypnotist may suggest that they no longer feel the urge to eat mindlessly or out of stress, and instead, feel empowered to make healthy choices that support their weight loss goals.

4. *Nail-Biting and Other Body-Focused Habits*

Nail-biting, hair-pulling, and other body-focused repetitive behaviors (BFRBs) are often rooted in anxiety, stress, or nervousness. These habits can be difficult to break because they are automatic and often go unnoticed. Hypnosis can help individuals become more aware of these behaviors and take control over them.

How Hypnosis Helps with Nail-Biting and BFRBs:

- *Identifying Triggers:* Hypnosis helps individuals become more aware of the emotional or environmental triggers that lead to the habit. Once these triggers are identified, the individual can be taught how to respond in healthier ways.
- *Reprogramming the Response:* Through suggestion, hypnosis helps the individual replace the automatic response of biting nails with a more positive behavior, such as taking a deep breath or tapping their fingers.
- *Boosting Self-Control and Awareness*: Hypnosis increases the individual's awareness of when they are engaging in the habit, helping them stop in the moment and redirect their behavior.
- *Reducing Anxiety:* Since many body-focused habits are linked to anxiety, hypnosis can help reduce the overall level of stress and anxiety, leading to a decrease in the frequency of these habits.

Example of Nail-Biting Technique:

- In a hypnosis session for nail-biting, the individual might be guided into a relaxed state and then given suggestions to associate nail-biting with an unpleasant sensation (like a bad taste or feeling) while introducing the idea that keeping hands clean or manicured feels better and more rewarding. Visualization techniques may also be used to imagine themselves with beautiful, healthy nails, reinforcing a new behavior.

5. *Overcoming Procrastination*

Procrastination is a habit that affects many people, causing them to delay important tasks, often due to fear of failure, perfectionism, or lack of motivation. Hypnosis can help break the cycle of procrastination by addressing the underlying causes and reprogramming the mind to take consistent action.

How Hypnosis Helps with Procrastination:

- *Identifying the Root Cause*: Hypnosis can help individuals uncover the emotional or psychological reasons behind their procrastination, whether it's fear of failure, perfectionism, or simply feeling overwhelmed by a task.
- *Reprogramming to Take Action:* Hypnosis works by reprogramming the subconscious mind to foster a sense of urgency and motivation. Suggestions for taking small steps toward completing a task are reinforced, making it easier to get started.
- *Increasing Self-Discipline:* Hypnosis can enhance self-discipline and willpower, encouraging the individual to prioritize their goals and take consistent action, even in the face of distractions or procrastination triggers.
- *Reducing Anxiety Around Tasks*: Often, procrastination is driven by anxiety related to starting or completing a task. Hypnosis can help reduce this anxiety, making the task feel more manageable and less intimidating.

Example of Procrastination Technique:

- A session for overcoming procrastination might involve using hypnosis to help the individual visualize completing a task successfully and effortlessly. The hypnotist may then provide suggestions that encourage taking immediate action, even on small steps, reinforcing a sense of accomplishment and progress.

Hypnosis is an effective and versatile tool for breaking bad habits and promoting healthier behaviors. Whether the habit involves smoking, overeating, nail-biting, procrastination, or other negative patterns, hypnosis works by accessing the subconscious mind and changing the automatic responses that drive these habits. By reprogramming the subconscious with positive suggestions, hypnosis makes it easier for individuals to adopt new, empowering behaviors that lead to lasting change. With dedication and support, hypnosis can help anyone overcome bad habits and create a healthier, more fulfilling lifestyle.

Hypnosis for Relaxation and Stress Relief: Methods for Helping Subjects Relax or Manage Stress

Stress is a pervasive challenge in modern life, impacting both mental and physical health. Chronic stress can lead to anxiety, insomnia, depression, and a host of physical ailments such as high blood pressure, heart disease, and digestive issues. One of the most effective and natural methods to combat stress is hypnosis, which facilitates deep relaxation and reprograms the mind to cope with stress in healthier ways. Hypnosis can help individuals break the cycle of stress, regain emotional balance, and promote physical well-being.

1. How Hypnosis Promotes Relaxation

Hypnosis induces a state of focused relaxation where the conscious mind is temporarily bypassed, and the subconscious mind is more receptive to calming suggestions. In this deeply relaxed state, the body and mind experience a reduction in stress, which can lead to numerous benefits including lowered anxiety, improved mood, and enhanced overall well-being.

Key Benefits of Hypnosis for Relaxation:

- *Inducing Deep Relaxation:* Hypnosis facilitates a deeply relaxed state by guiding the individual into a calm, peaceful mental and physical state. This process can include controlled breathing, muscle relaxation, and calming imagery.
- *Reducing Physical Symptoms of Stress:* During hypnosis, individuals experience reduced heart rate, slower breathing, and lower blood pressure—physiological markers that signal relaxation and stress relief. This helps reverse the harmful effects of chronic stress on the body.

- *Releasing Tension:* Hypnosis can guide individuals to focus on relaxing specific muscle groups, releasing built-up tension in the body. This can be particularly effective for those who carry stress in areas such as the neck, shoulders, or jaw.
- *Promoting Mental Calmness*: Hypnosis encourages the individual to clear their mind of racing thoughts and worries, helping them focus on peaceful, calming sensations or images. This mental calmness helps counteract feelings of overwhelm and anxiety.

2. Relaxation Techniques in Hypnosis

Several techniques within hypnosis are specifically designed to promote relaxation and stress relief. These techniques are often used in combination or can be adapted based on the individual's needs.

Key Hypnotic Relaxation Techniques:

- *Progressive Relaxation:* Progressive relaxation is one of the most common techniques used in hypnosis for relaxation. It involves guiding the individual to focus on different parts of their body, beginning with the feet and moving upwards, encouraging each muscle group to relax and release tension. This technique helps the individual become more aware of where they are holding tension and teaches them how to consciously release it.
    - *How It Works:* The hypnotist suggests that the individual relax each body part in sequence, such as: "Now, let your feet feel completely relaxed, as though they are sinking into the ground. Allow the muscles in your legs to release any tension..."
    - *Example*: A common variation of progressive relaxation is to use mental imagery alongside it. The individual might imagine their stress melting away like ice under the sun as they move through the different muscle groups.
- *Breathing Techniques:* Deep, controlled breathing is an integral part of hypnosis. Slow, deep breaths stimulate the parasympathetic nervous system, which induces the body's "relaxation response." Breathing techniques can be combined with hypnotic suggestions to

encourage calmness and release stress.

- *How It Works:* The hypnotist may guide the subject to breathe in slowly through the nose for a count of four, hold the breath for four seconds, and then exhale slowly through the mouth. This process can be repeated, with each exhalation helping to release tension and calm the mind.
- *Example*: "With every breath, you feel more relaxed, more at ease. As you breathe in, you feel calmness entering your body, and as you exhale, you release any remaining stress."

- *Visualization and Guided Imagery:* Visualization is a powerful tool in hypnosis. The subject is guided to imagine relaxing scenes or environments—such as a peaceful beach, a quiet forest, or a serene mountain top. These mental images evoke feelings of calmness and tranquility, helping the individual disconnect from stressors in their life.

  - *How It Works:* The hypnotist guides the subject to vividly imagine a peaceful place, encouraging them to focus on the details—like the sound of waves on the shore, the scent of pine trees, or the warmth of the sun on their skin.
  - *Example*: "Imagine you are walking along a peaceful beach. The soft sand feels warm under your feet. The gentle sound of the waves soothes you, and the cool breeze refreshes you. With each step, you feel lighter and more relaxed."

- *Self-Hypnosis for Relaxation*: Self-hypnosis is a valuable tool that individuals can use outside of formal hypnosis sessions to manage stress on their own. Through self-hypnosis, the individual learns to relax deeply and focus their attention in ways that release tension and foster a calm, centered state.

  - *How It Works:* Self-hypnosis typically involves creating a calm, quiet environment, using relaxation techniques, and repeating calming phrases or mantras. The individual can also use guided imagery to promote relaxation.
  - *Example*: "I am calm, centered, and at peace. I feel the stress melting away with every breath I take. My body is relaxed, and my mind is quiet."

3. Stress Relief through Hypnosis

Hypnosis helps to alleviate stress by reducing the physical and emotional symptoms of anxiety and tension. While relaxation techniques are key to stress relief, hypnosis also works on the deeper, underlying causes of stress, such as negative thought patterns, fear, or unresolved emotions.

How Hypnosis Reduces Stress:

- *Addressing the Root Cause of Stress:* Hypnosis can uncover and address the subconscious triggers that contribute to stress. For example, unresolved trauma, excessive worry, or perfectionistic tendencies may be identified and reframed during hypnosis, helping the individual cope with stress in a healthier way.
- *Shifting Negative Thought Patterns:* Often, stress is caused by negative thinking—such as catastrophic thinking, excessive worry, or self-doubt. Hypnosis can help shift these thought patterns by providing suggestions that replace negative thoughts with more balanced and positive perspectives.
    - *Example*: The hypnotist might suggest, "You now choose to respond to challenges with calmness and clarity. You know that you are capable of handling whatever comes your way with confidence and ease."
- *Relaxing the Body's Stress Response:* Hypnosis can be used to alter the body's automatic stress response. Through suggestions of calmness, the hypnotist helps the body release physical tension, reduce the production of stress hormones like cortisol, and encourage the production of feel-good chemicals such as endorphins.
    - *Example*: "Your body is learning to respond to stress in a more relaxed, balanced way. You are releasing all the tension in your muscles, and with every breath, your body is becoming more and more relaxed."
- *Reframing Stressful Situations*: Through hypnosis, individuals can learn to reframe situations that might normally cause them stress. For instance, what might have been perceived as a threat or overwhelming challenge can be viewed through a different lens, enabling the person to manage their emotional response more effectively.

◦ *Example*: "You now see challenges as opportunities for growth, not threats. You trust that you are capable of handling any situation that comes your way, and you feel confident in your ability to cope."

4. Stress Management for Specific Situations

Hypnosis can also be targeted to help individuals manage stress in specific situations, such as:

- *Work-related Stress:* Hypnosis can be used to reduce stress at work by helping individuals manage deadlines, interpersonal conflicts, or feelings of overwhelm. Techniques like visualization can be used to promote a sense of calm during stressful meetings or presentations.
    - ◦ *Example*: "Imagine yourself at work, handling tasks effortlessly and with focus. You are confident, calm, and in control, no matter what the day brings."
- *Public Speaking Anxiety*: Many individuals experience stress related to public speaking. Hypnosis can help reduce anxiety before and during presentations by calming the body, shifting thoughts away from fear, and promoting positive self-talk.
    - ◦ *Example*: "When you step onto the stage, you feel confident and composed. You focus on delivering your message with clarity, and you enjoy the experience of speaking to your audience."
- *Sleep-Related Stress:* Stress often affects sleep quality, leading to insomnia or disturbed sleep. Hypnosis can promote relaxation and reduce stress-related sleep issues by encouraging the body to unwind and enter a peaceful, restful state.
    - ◦ *Example*: "As you lay in bed, your body is relaxed, and your mind is calm. You feel a wave of relaxation wash over you, and soon, you drift off into a deep, restful sleep."

Hypnosis is a highly effective tool for relaxation and stress relief. By accessing the subconscious mind, hypnosis helps individuals manage and reduce stress by promoting relaxation, reprogramming negative thought patterns, and addressing the underlying causes of anxiety and tension. Through techniques like progressive relaxation, guided imagery, and deep breathing, hypnosis offers a natural, sustainable way to cope with stress and maintain emotional and physical well-being. Whether used for general relaxation or targeted stress management in specific situations, hypnosis can be an invaluable tool for anyone looking to reduce stress and improve their quality of life.

Chapter 9: Advanced Techniques

Fragment Therapy: Using Hypnosis to Address Internal Conflicts or Multiple Aspects of a Person's Psyche

I coined the term "Fragment Therapy" in 1992 to signify an advanced hypnosis technique that delves deep into the subconscious to address internal conflicts, contradictions, or unresolved issues within a person's psyche. It is based on the idea that an individual's mind is composed of different "Fragments" or "subpersonalities" that represent various emotional, behavioral, or cognitive states. These fragments often manifest in the form of inner conflicts, such as a person wanting to quit a bad habit but feeling a powerful urge to continue it, or desiring success but subconsciously sabotaging their progress. Fragment Therapy uses hypnosis to identify, communicate with, and harmonize these Fragments, leading to personal integration and healing.

1. Understanding Fragment Therapy

In Fragment Therapy, the mind is viewed as a collection of fragments, each of which has a specific function or role. These fragments might represent desires, fears, values, or unresolved emotional experiences that influence behavior and mental health. Often, these fragments conflict with one another, leading to feelings of confusion, frustration, or inner turmoil. For example, one fragment might want to succeed and take action, while another fragment may be afraid of failure and procrastinates. The goal of Fragment Therapy is to help these fragments communicate and work together harmoniously, eliminating the internal conflicts that create emotional and behavioral problems.

Key Concepts of Fragment Therapy:

- *Fragment of the Psyche:* These fragments are distinct aspects of a person's consciousness that may represent emotions, desires, beliefs, or coping mechanisms. Fragments may be conscious (e.g., the rational aspect of the mind) or subconscious (e.g., the aspect of the mind holding past trauma or unresolved emotions).

- *Internal Conflicts:* Conflicts arise when different fragments of the psyche want different things or hold opposing beliefs. For instance, someone might want to quit smoking (a healthy aspect of the mind), but another aspect of the mind might still crave the habit (a fear or coping mechanism).
- *Inner Dialogue:* Fragment Therapy involves facilitating dialogue between different fragments of the psyche to understand their perspectives, negotiate, and resolve internal conflicts.
- *Integration*: The ultimate aim of Fragment Therapy is integration, where all fragments of the psyche are aligned and working together for the individual's best interest.

2. The Role of Hypnosis in Fragment Therapy

Hypnosis can play a crucial role in Fragment Therapy by allowing the individual to enter a deeply relaxed, receptive state in which they can access the subconscious fragment of their mind. In this relaxed state, the person can identify, communicate with, and facilitate positive change within the conflicting fragment of their psyche. The hypnotist guides the individual through the process of communicating with different fragments, helping them to resolve conflicts and align the fragment with the person's goals.

How Hypnosis Enhances Fragment Therapy:

- *Accessing the Subconscious:* Hypnosis bypasses the conscious mind, which is often resistant to change, and allows the individual to access deeper levels of the subconscious, where the fragment resides.
- *Facilitating Dialogue*: During hypnosis, the hypnotist helps the individual communicate with different fragments of their psyche, providing a safe and controlled environment for these fragments to express their concerns, needs, and desires.
- *Reframing Beliefs:* Hypnosis can reframe limiting beliefs held by conflicting fragments. For example, if one aspect is afraid of failure, hypnosis can guide that fragment to understand that failure is not

dangerous and that growth comes from learning.

- *Creating Internal Harmony*: The hypnotist uses suggestions and visualization to promote understanding and harmony between fragments, ensuring that they work together in support of the individual's greater well-being and goals.

3. Steps in Fragment Therapy

Fragment Therapy typically follows a structured process that allows the individual to explore and integrate the different fragments of their psyche. The hypnotist facilitates this process by guiding the subject into a relaxed state and then working through the steps outlined below.

Step 1: Induction and Relaxation

The session begins with the hypnotist guiding the individual into a relaxed, trance-like state. The hypnotist uses progressive relaxation or other techniques to help the subject become deeply relaxed, creating a receptive state for accessing the subconscious mind.

Step 2: Identifying the Fragment

Once the person is in a relaxed state, the hypnotist helps them identify the conflicting fragments within their psyche. The individual may be asked to focus on the specific issue or challenge they are facing (e.g., quitting smoking, overcoming procrastination, or managing anxiety) and become aware of the different fragments involved.

- *Example*: "As you focus on your desire to quit smoking, what aspect of you wants to quit, and what aspect of you resists that decision? Notice how these fragments feel and what they represent."

Step 3: Communicating with the Fragment

After identifying the fragment, the hypnotist guides the subject in initiating a dialogue between them. Each fragment is given the opportunity to speak and express its intentions, fears, desires, and concerns. The hypnotist helps the subject listen actively to each fragment, fostering an understanding of their roles and motivations.

- *Example*: "Now, let the fragment that wants you to quit smoking speak. What does this fragment want? What does it need to feel safe and supported in making this change?"

- *Example*: "Now, let the fragment that resists quitting speak. What are its concerns? What does it fear might happen if you stop smoking?"

Step 4: Resolving Conflict and Negotiating

Once the fragments have communicated, the hypnotist helps the individual facilitate a resolution to the conflict. The goal is to create a dialogue where the fragments feel heard and understood. Often, this involves reframing the negative beliefs or emotions held by the resisting fragment, helping it realize that its original purpose (e.g., providing comfort or coping with stress) can be met in healthier ways.

- *Example*: "What if the fragment that resists quitting smoking could find another way to feel relaxed and safe? Perhaps it could support you in developing new habits or coping strategies."
- *Example*: "How can the fragment that wants you to quit smoking assure the resisting fragment that the change will bring more freedom and health, without feeling deprived or threatened?"

Step 5: Integration and Healing

Once the fragments have resolved their conflict, the hypnotist works to integrate them, creating a new internal harmony. The conflicting fragments are encouraged to work together to support the individual's overall goals. This integration often results in feelings of wholeness and increased mental clarity.

- *Example*: "Now that the fragments have come to an agreement, imagine them joining together, working in unity to support your well-being. Visualize the changes that you will experience as you work in alignment with yourself."

Step 6: Post-Hypnotic Suggestions

To reinforce the integration, the hypnotist offers post-hypnotic suggestions that help the individual continue to experience internal harmony after the session. These suggestions might include reminders of the new cooperation between fragments or reinforcement of the newly learned coping strategies.

- *Example*: "From now on, whenever you encounter stress, the fragments that once conflicted will work together to find a solution that is healthy and supportive. You feel calm, centered, and in control."

4. Benefits of Fragment Therapy

Fragment Therapy offers several benefits for individuals looking to resolve internal conflicts and gain greater emotional and mental stability. Some of the key benefits include:

Increased Self-Awareness:

Fragment Therapy encourages individuals to explore and understand the different fragments of themselves, leading to a deeper awareness of their emotional and psychological landscape. This awareness helps individuals recognize how internal conflicts influence their behaviors and decisions.

Conflict Resolution:

By resolving inner conflicts, Fragment Therapy helps individuals align their thoughts, emotions, and behaviors. This leads to increased emotional balance, reduced anxiety, and a greater sense of self-acceptance.

Improved Decision-Making:

Once the conflicting fragments are harmonized, individuals are better equipped to make decisions that align with their true desires and goals, free from the internal tug-of-war that often leads to indecision and procrastination.

Healing Past Wounds:

Fragment Therapy can help individuals address unresolved emotional wounds by communicating with the fragment that holds onto past trauma. Healing these wounds can lead to greater emotional freedom and mental well-being.

Empowered Change:

By integrating the conflicting fragments, Fragment Therapy empowers individuals to make lasting changes. When the psyche is working in harmony, behavior change becomes easier, and the person is better equipped to handle future challenges.

Fragment Therapy is a powerful advanced hypnosis technique that helps individuals resolve internal conflicts, harmonize different aspects of their psyche, and promote emotional healing. By accessing the subconscious mind, hypnosis allows individuals to communicate with and integrate various fragments of themselves, addressing the root causes of inner tension and facilitating lasting change. Whether the conflict arises from emotional wounds, negative beliefs, or sabotaging behaviors, Fragment Therapy offers a pathway to self-awareness, personal growth, and healing. If you are interested in self-healing, please read my book: *Telman Fragment Therapy: A Complete Guide to Self-Healing*.

Age Regression: A Technique for Revisiting Past Memories for Healing or Understanding

Age Regression is a therapeutic technique in hypnosis that involves guiding an individual back in time to revisit earlier experiences or past memories, often to gain insight, resolve emotional issues, or heal unresolved trauma. It is based on the idea that certain memories and emotional patterns from the past—particularly from childhood or earlier life—can continue to influence a person's present behavior, emotions, and mental well-being. By accessing and processing these memories in a safe, controlled environment, individuals can achieve emotional healing, gain understanding, and release old, limiting beliefs or traumas that may be hindering their growth or happiness.

1. Understanding Age Regression

Age Regression is a form of deep hypnosis where the subject is guided to mentally regress to an earlier point in their life. The goal of this technique is to explore memories, emotions, and experiences that may not be consciously remembered, but which still influence current thoughts, behaviors, and emotional states. It is often used for therapeutic purposes, such as uncovering the roots of phobias, anxieties, trauma, or unexplained emotional reactions.

While in a regressed state, the individual may experience memories and emotions from their past, often with a new perspective, allowing them to process and heal unresolved issues. This can be particularly useful for understanding the origins of current behaviors or patterns, such as fear, self-sabotage, or recurring relationship problems.

2. How Age Regression Works in Hypnosis

In a typical Age Regression session, the hypnotist induces a deep trance state and then guides the individual back in time to a specific memory or time in their life. The process involves using various techniques to help the person access their subconscious mind, bypassing the critical conscious mind and allowing the individual to retrieve memories, both conscious and subconscious. These memories can range from recent past experiences to deeply buried childhood memories or even past life experiences, depending on the type of regression used.

Key Concepts of Age Regression:

- *Subconscious Mind Access:* The subconscious mind stores memories, emotions, and experiences that are not always readily accessible through conscious thought. Hypnosis helps bypass the conscious mind and connect directly with these deeper layers of memory.
- *Guided Exploration:* The hypnotist guides the subject to specific points in their past, encouraging them to relive and process memories. This exploration can occur in stages, with the subject revisiting different times or experiences in their life.
- *Memory Recollection:* The process may evoke vivid memories, sensory experiences, emotions, and sensations, all of which are used to gain deeper insights into current issues or conflicts.

Age Regression Process:

- *Induction into Hypnosis:* The subject is guided into a deep state of relaxation using standard hypnotic techniques such as progressive relaxation, deep breathing, or visualization.
- *Regression to Childhood*: Once the person is deeply relaxed, the hypnotist guides them to imagine or mentally move backward in time, beginning with their most recent memory and then progressively moving further back in time. The individual may be asked to visualize specific ages or times in their life.
- *Exploring Memories:* As the subject revisits past memories, they may experience thoughts, emotions, and sensations associated with those times. The hypnotist encourages the subject to observe and process these memories in a safe, supportive way.
- *Therapeutic Processing*: The hypnotist may use techniques such as reframing, suggestion, or emotional release to help the individual

process the emotions or beliefs tied to these memories. This helps the person release any emotional baggage or limiting beliefs carried from the past.

3. Applications of Age Regression

Age Regression can be used for a variety of therapeutic purposes, from addressing unresolved trauma to understanding the origins of emotional patterns. Some common applications include:

1. Trauma Healing

One of the most powerful uses of Age Regression is in healing past trauma. Many traumatic experiences, especially those from childhood, can have long-lasting effects on an individual's mental health. By regressing to the memory of the traumatic event, the person can experience it with a new perspective and in a safe, controlled environment. This process helps to release the emotional charge tied to the event, allowing for healing.

- *Example*: A person who has a fear of speaking in public might have experienced humiliation or embarrassment during childhood that led to this phobia. Age Regression can allow them to revisit and process the original experience, which can diminish the intensity of the fear.

2. Resolving Emotional Blockages

Sometimes, people experience emotions or behaviors that seem to come from nowhere—such as unexplained anger, anxiety, or sadness. These feelings are often rooted in past experiences or unresolved emotional conflicts. By exploring early memories through Age Regression, individuals can discover the origins of these emotions and gain insights that allow them to release these blockages.

- *Example*: Someone who has difficulty trusting others may uncover early childhood experiences where they were betrayed by a caregiver or experienced abandonment. By processing these memories, they may be able to let go of old fears and rebuild trust.

3. Overcoming Limiting Beliefs

Many of the beliefs we hold about ourselves and the world are formed during childhood. Negative experiences can lead to beliefs like "I'm not good enough" or "I can't succeed." Age Regression can be used to identify the origins of these beliefs and reframe them, leading to improved self-esteem and a healthier mindset.

- *Example*: A person who constantly fears failure might uncover memories of being criticized or judged harshly in school. By reinterpreting these experiences through Age Regression, they can begin to release these limiting beliefs and replace them with more empowering ones.

4. Exploring Past Lives (Past Life Regression)

Some practitioners of Age Regression also use the technique to explore past lives. While controversial and not universally accepted, past life regression involves guiding the individual to experience memories of a past life, with the goal of understanding their current issues from a broader perspective. People who believe in reincarnation may find this approach helpful in exploring patterns or unresolved issues that seem to transcend their current life.

- *Example*: Someone with a recurring fear of water may uncover a memory of drowning in a past life, which provides insight into their current fear and offers a path for healing.

5. Understanding Current Patterns and Behaviors

Age Regression can be an effective way to uncover the root causes of present-day behaviors or issues. This technique can help individuals understand why they react in certain ways to specific situations and offer them the opportunity to rewrite old patterns that no longer serve them.

- *Example*: A person who struggles with relationships might use Age Regression to uncover early memories of attachment or abandonment issues that shaped their adult relationships. Understanding these patterns can lead to healthier relationship dynamics in the present.

4. Techniques Used in Age Regression

Several techniques can be used during an Age Regression session to enhance the experience and ensure a safe and effective process:

- *Time Travel Technique:* The hypnotist guides the individual to mentally travel back in time to specific ages or stages of life. The subject may be asked to visualize walking down a staircase or traveling in a balloon as they move backward through time.
    - *Example*: "As you relax, imagine you are standing at the top of a staircase. With each number I say, you will move down one step, going back in time. Ten... nine... eight... until we reach the age where we want to begin our journey."
- *Age Regression to Specific Memories:* The subject is asked to regress to a specific event or memory, such as a childhood trauma, to re-experience and process the emotional impact of that event.
    - *Example*: "Let's go back to a time when you first experienced fear. Can you bring up that memory? Allow yourself to experience it fully, and notice what it feels like now from your current perspective."
- *Reframing and Healing:* Once the memory is accessed, the hypnotist may guide the person to reframe the experience or offer new, empowering suggestions. This could involve allowing the individual to interact with their younger self, offering love, support, or comfort that they might not have received at the time.
    - *Example*: "Now, as you revisit that difficult moment, imagine your adult self stepping in to comfort your younger self. What would you say to them to help them feel safe and supported?"
- *Positive Suggestions and Empowerment:* To ensure the individual leaves the session feeling empowered and healed, positive suggestions are used to help them embrace new beliefs and behaviors.
    - *Example*: "From now on, you will remember this event as a turning point in your life, one where you became stronger and more resilient. You are safe, supported, and capable of handling any challenge that comes your way."

5. Benefits of Age Regression

Age Regression offers numerous benefits, including:

- *Emotional Healing:* By revisiting and processing past traumatic events, individuals can heal from emotional wounds that have been affecting them for years.

- *Increased Self-Understanding:* Age Regression allows individuals to gain deeper insight into their behaviors, emotions, and patterns, leading to greater self-awareness.
- *Releasing Limiting Beliefs*: The technique helps individuals identify and release negative beliefs formed in childhood or earlier years that are holding them back from reaching their potential.
- *Resolution of Fears and Phobias: By* uncovering the root causes of irrational fears or phobias, individuals can gain the clarity and emotional release needed to overcome them.
- *Improved Relationships:* Addressing early attachment issues or unresolved childhood traumas can lead to healthier, more balanced relationships in adulthood.

Age Regression is a powerful therapeutic technique that uses hypnosis to revisit past memories for healing, understanding, and self-awareness. By accessing the subconscious mind and exploring significant events in one's life, individuals can uncover the roots of their current emotional struggles and behavioral patterns. Through the process of revisiting and reframing these experiences, individuals can heal past wounds, release limiting beliefs, and achieve a greater sense of emotional balance and personal growth.

Reframing and Cognitive Restructuring: Techniques for Changing Thought Patterns Through Hypnosis

Reframing and cognitive restructuring are therapeutic techniques used to alter negative or unhelpful thought patterns and replace them with more constructive, positive alternatives. In hypnosis, these techniques become even more powerful, as the relaxed and focused state allows access to the subconscious mind, where many of these thought patterns are rooted. By using hypnosis to guide individuals in reframing their perspectives, it is possible to create lasting changes in the way they think, feel, and behave.

1. Understanding Reframing and Cognitive Restructuring

Reframing

Reframing involves changing the way an individual perceives or interprets a situation, event, or experience. The goal is to shift the emotional charge or belief associated with that experience. It doesn't necessarily change the event itself, but it alters how the individual thinks about and responds to it. Reframing often involves helping the person see a situation from a different perspective, allowing them to view it in a more positive or neutral light.

Cognitive Restructuring

Cognitive restructuring is a technique that involves identifying and challenging irrational or distorted thought patterns and replacing them with more balanced and rational thoughts. This process helps individuals overcome cognitive distortions like all-or-nothing thinking, catastrophizing, or overgeneralization, which can contribute to anxiety, depression, and other emotional difficulties. Both reframing and cognitive restructuring aim to break the cycle of negative thinking, reduce emotional distress, and improve overall mental health by empowering individuals to think differently.

2. The Role of Hypnosis in Reframing and Cognitive Restructuring

Hypnosis can enhance the process of reframing and cognitive restructuring by accessing the subconscious mind, where deeply ingrained thought patterns and beliefs often reside. In a relaxed, focused state, individuals are more open to suggestions and able to process emotional material more effectively. This makes hypnosis a powerful tool for shifting perceptions, challenging limiting beliefs, and promoting lasting change.

- *Accessing the Subconscious Mind:* In hypnosis, the conscious mind is less active, allowing the subconscious mind to become more accessible. Since most negative thought patterns or cognitive distortions are stored in the subconscious, hypnosis allows these thought patterns to be addressed at their root.
- *Increased Suggestibility:* The heightened suggestibility of the hypnotic state enables individuals to accept new, healthier thought patterns more easily, especially when these suggestions are framed in a way

that feels natural and congruent with their values.

- *Relaxation and Emotional Releasing:* Hypnosis induces a deep state of relaxation, which can help individuals process emotions that are tied to negative thoughts. Emotional release is often an important part of reframing or restructuring thought patterns, as it allows individuals to let go of old emotional baggage that may have influenced their thinking.

3. Techniques for Reframing and Cognitive Restructuring in Hypnosis

Here are some specific techniques for reframing and cognitive restructuring that can be used within a hypnotic context:

1. Positive Reframing

In this technique, the hypnotist helps the subject change their perspective on a situation by finding a positive or neutral aspect in an otherwise negative event or belief. For example, if a person perceives failure as a personal deficiency, the hypnotist may guide them to reframe failure as a valuable learning experience.

- *Example*: "In the past, you may have viewed mistakes or failures as negative experiences. But now, you realize that each of these experiences is an opportunity to learn, grow, and improve. Mistakes are simply stepping stones toward your success."

2. Visualization of Alternative Perspectives

Using vivid imagery, the hypnotist guides the person to imagine themselves in a situation but with a new, more positive interpretation. The individual might be asked to imagine how they would behave or feel in the situation if they had a more empowering belief or thought.

- *Example*: "Imagine the last time you faced a challenging situation. Now, picture yourself handling that situation with calm and confidence. See yourself making clear decisions, feeling strong, and knowing that you can handle whatever comes your way. Notice how different your experience is when you view it from this empowered perspective."

3. Cognitive Restructuring through Questioning

The hypnotist can guide the subject to challenge their negative thought patterns by asking thought-provoking questions. This technique helps the individual examine the validity of their beliefs and recognize distortions in their thinking. Through hypnosis, the person is in a more relaxed and open state, making them more receptive to questioning and challenging their assumptions.

- *Example*: "What evidence do you have that supports the thought that you are not good enough? Can you think of past situations where you succeeded, even when you didn't feel perfect? What alternative, more helpful thoughts can you adopt instead of that negative belief?"

4. Substitution of Negative Thoughts with Positive Affirmations

During hypnosis, the hypnotist may guide the person to replace negative or irrational thoughts with positive, empowering affirmations. These affirmations are carefully crafted to challenge the old beliefs and encourage new, healthier ways of thinking.

- *Example*: "Whenever you feel that negative thought creeping in, you can replace it with, 'I am capable, I am worthy, and I handle challenges with ease.' You now have the ability to automatically replace old, unhelpful thoughts with empowering beliefs that align with your goals."

5. Anchoring Positive States

Anchoring is a technique used in hypnosis to create a mental association between a certain physical gesture, word, or image and a positive emotional state. By anchoring a positive feeling to a specific trigger, the person can use that anchor in everyday life to reinforce their new cognitive patterns.

- *Example*: "As you relax deeply, you can imagine yourself experiencing a time when you felt completely confident and calm. Now, as you tap your fingers together, that feeling of confidence will be anchored in your mind. The next time you face a difficult situation, you can use this anchor to bring back that calm and positive mindset."

4. Overcoming Cognitive Distortions through Hypnosis

Cognitive distortions are irrational or exaggerated thought patterns that can negatively impact mental health. Hypnosis can be an effective tool for identifying and challenging these distortions. Here are some common cognitive distortions and how hypnosis can be used to address them:

1. All-or-Nothing Thinking

This distortion involves viewing situations in extremes, such as seeing something as either completely good or completely bad, with no middle ground. Hypnosis can help the individual recognize this pattern and practice seeing situations from a more balanced perspective.

- *Example*: "When you catch yourself thinking that something is either all good or all bad, pause and ask yourself, 'Is there any middle ground here? What are some positive aspects of this situation that I may not be seeing?'"

2. Catastrophizing

Catastrophizing involves expecting the worst-case scenario, even in situations where it's unlikely. In hypnosis, the person can be guided to challenge these worst-case scenarios and reframe them in a more realistic, grounded way.

- *Example*: "When you find yourself imagining the worst possible outcome, take a moment to ask yourself, 'What is the most likely outcome, and how can I prepare for it in a calm and effective way?'"

3. Overgeneralization

This distortion involves making broad conclusions based on a single event. Hypnosis can help the person see that one isolated experience does not define their entire life or future.

- *Example*: "When you find yourself thinking that one mistake means you will always fail, challenge that belief by asking, 'Can I think of any examples where I succeeded after facing setbacks?'"

4. Personalization

Personalization is when a person takes responsibility for events outside their control, often leading to unnecessary guilt or self-blame. Hypnosis can help the individual reframe these beliefs and accept responsibility where it's due, while letting go of what they cannot control.

- *Example*: "If you ever find yourself blaming yourself for things that were beyond your control, remind yourself, 'I am responsible for my actions, but there are many factors I cannot control. I can let go of unnecessary guilt and focus on what I can change.'"

5. Benefits of Reframing and Cognitive Restructuring in Hypnosis

- *Improved Emotional Well-Being:* By changing negative thought patterns, individuals experience reduced anxiety, depression, and emotional distress.
- *Increased Self-Efficacy:* Reframing and restructuring thought patterns empower individuals to feel more in control of their lives, boosting confidence and self-belief.
- *Enhanced Problem-Solving*: Shifting perspectives can help individuals view challenges as opportunities, making them more resilient and resourceful in the face of adversity.
- *Long-Term Change:* Because hypnosis works with the subconscious mind, changes in thought patterns are often more profound and lasting compared to conventional cognitive-behavioral methods alone.

Reframing and cognitive restructuring are potent techniques for changing thought patterns and creating lasting positive change. Through hypnosis, individuals can access the subconscious mind, where negative beliefs and cognitive distortions are often stored. By using specific techniques like positive reframing, visualization, and thought substitution, individuals can challenge and replace limiting beliefs with empowering ones. The result is improved emotional well-being, increased self-confidence, and a greater ability to manage life's challenges with a positive, resilient mindset.

Confusion and Ericksonian Methods: Using Confusion and Conversational Hypnosis to Induce Trance

Confusion techniques and Ericksonian hypnosis are powerful methods used to induce hypnosis in a more subtle and indirect way, relying on conversational patterns, ambiguity, and disorientation to guide individuals into a trance state. These methods can be especially useful in situations where direct induction techniques might not be appropriate, or when a more conversational, natural approach is desired. In this section, we will explore how confusion and Ericksonian methods can be used effectively for trance induction and therapeutic purposes.

1. Understanding Confusion Techniques

Confusion techniques are based on the principle of cognitive disorientation. By introducing an element of confusion into a conversation, the hypnotist can disrupt the subject's normal thought patterns, creating a gap in their mental processing. This gap makes the individual more suggestible and open to entering a trance state.

When the conscious mind is confused or distracted, it becomes less dominant, allowing the subconscious mind to take the lead. This opens the door to more effective suggestion and deeper hypnotic states. Confusion techniques often involve paradoxical language, ambiguous phrasing, and complex ideas that require the person's focus and attention to process. As the person becomes mentally engaged in trying to make sense of the confusion, they become more receptive to hypnotic suggestions.

How Confusion Induces Trance

- *Cognitive Overload:* Introducing multiple ideas or concepts in rapid succession causes the conscious mind to experience a temporary overload. The subconscious mind steps in to make sense of the chaos, facilitating relaxation and openness to suggestion.
- *Indirect Communication:* Through indirect language patterns, the hypnotist can confuse the subject into letting go of resistance and logical analysis, making them more susceptible to hypnotic influence.
- *Disruption of Normal Thinking:* A sudden shift in thought or conversation can cause the individual to pause, creating a moment of

mental "blankness" where the subconscious mind becomes more active.

2. Ericksonian Hypnosis and Conversational Techniques

Ericksonian hypnosis, developed by Dr. Milton H. Erickson, is a form of indirect hypnosis that emphasizes the use of language, storytelling, and metaphor to facilitate trance and therapeutic change. Dr. Erickson was known for using conversational hypnosis, which involves integrating hypnotic language into normal conversation without the subject even realizing they are being hypnotized.

Key Principles of Ericksonian Methods

- *Utilization*: The hypnotist uses whatever the subject brings to the session—whether thoughts, behaviors, or attitudes—as a means to facilitate the hypnotic process. This makes the technique highly adaptable and tailored to the individual.
- *Metaphors and Stories*: Erickson frequently used metaphors, anecdotes, and stories to bypass the subject's critical mind and communicate directly with the subconscious. These stories often contain embedded suggestions that lead to therapeutic outcomes.
- *Ambiguity*: Erickson often used ambiguous language, leaving room for multiple interpretations. This causes the conscious mind to become uncertain, allowing the subconscious mind to engage with the hypnotic suggestion on a deeper level.
- *Pacing and Leading*: This technique involves first matching (pacing) the person's current state or behavior and then gradually leading them toward a new, desired state. The hypnotist builds rapport by aligning with the person's experience before gently guiding them toward trance.

3. Using Confusion to Induce Trance

Confusion methods, especially in the context of Ericksonian hypnosis, often involve a series of techniques designed to disrupt the subject's usual mental processes and induce a trance state.

Confusion Techniques:

- *Double Binds:* A double bind presents the subject with two equally valid options, making them feel compelled to choose one, even though both options lead to the same outcome. This confusion helps bypass critical thinking and opens the door to deeper mental processing.
    - *Example*: "Would you prefer to relax deeply now, or would you prefer to relax deeply in a moment?" This ambiguity causes the person to engage their subconscious mind to resolve the confusion, leading them into trance.
- *Rapid, Shifting Language*: Speaking rapidly or shifting between topics, especially when the ideas are somewhat unrelated or contradictory, can cause cognitive overload, making it easier for the subject to let go of logical thinking and enter a trance.
    - *Example*: "And as you listen to my voice now, you might find that you're becoming more and more relaxed, or perhaps, you're thinking about something completely unrelated, like a memory from years ago... but then again, that's not what matters right now."
- *Paradoxical Statements:* Paradoxical statements create cognitive dissonance by offering two contradictory ideas at the same time, forcing the individual to let go of their usual analytical mindset and accept the paradox as it is. This can confuse the conscious mind and allow the subconscious to take control.
    - *Example*: "You might not even realize how deeply relaxed you are becoming, or perhaps you're already aware of it. Either way, it's happening, isn't it?"
- *Overloading with Information:* Providing an excess of information or sensory input can be overwhelming for the conscious mind, allowing the subconscious to take over. The hypnotist may tell stories, offer descriptions, or use words in ways that don't follow logical sequences, further confusing the subject.
    - *Example*: "Notice how the temperature in the room changes, and maybe you're aware of the sound of my voice, but perhaps there's a slight

rustling in the air, or even the sound of your breath, which could feel different than usual. As you think about all these sensations, your mind might find a way to relax even more, and you may not even know exactly when you become so deeply relaxed."

4. Conversational Hypnosis: Subtle Techniques for Inducing Trance

Conversational hypnosis relies heavily on language patterns that subtly guide the subject into a trance without overt suggestion. Ericksonian techniques are often employed in everyday interactions, making them ideal for situations where overt hypnotic inductions are not practical or desirable.

Techniques of Conversational Hypnosis:

- *Pacing and Leading:* The hypnotist first mirrors the subject's current state (pacing), then gently leads them to a more relaxed or suggestible state. The hypnotist may mirror body language, breathing patterns, or tone of voice to build rapport and trust.
  - *Example:* "As you're sitting comfortably there, breathing in and out, just like you have been all this time, you might notice how easy it is to let go, to simply follow my voice and relax deeper with each breath."
- *Embedded Commands*: Commands are embedded within normal conversation, often in the form of suggestions that are disguised within longer sentences. These commands are typically imperceptible to the conscious mind, allowing them to be absorbed by the subconscious.
  - *Example*: "You can begin to relax more deeply, and as you relax, you might find that you can let go of tension easily, or perhaps, notice how your body just naturally becomes more comfortable with every passing moment."
- *The Use of "Maybe" and "Perhaps":* These words create uncertainty, allowing the subject's subconscious mind to fill in the blanks with the desired outcome. These words invite the subject to participate in the hypnotic process without feeling forced.
  - *Example*: "Maybe, as you listen to my voice, you'll start to notice that your body feels heavier, perhaps more relaxed, or maybe you'll just feel a

sense of calm washing over you… either way, that's fine."

- *Interrupting the Pattern:* By interrupting a person's usual pattern of thinking or speaking, the hypnotist creates an opening for the subconscious to take over. This can be achieved by changing the subject, using unexpected statements, or even pausing in conversation to give the subject time to process and slip into a trance.
  - *Example*: "And as you're thinking about that, you might also start to realize how deep your breath is, or maybe how calm you're starting to feel. It's interesting, isn't it?"

5. Benefits and Applications of Confusion and Ericksonian Methods

- *Subtle Trance Induction:* These methods allow the hypnotist to induce trance without the subject realizing it, making them ideal for situations where overt hypnosis is not appropriate (e.g., in public or therapeutic settings).
- *Increased Suggestibility:* Confusion and Ericksonian methods work well to make the subject more open to suggestion and change, as the conscious mind becomes distracted and less focused on analyzing or resisting the process.
- *Effective for Resistance:* These methods can be particularly useful when working with resistant subjects, as they bypass the critical, conscious mind and create opportunities for the subconscious to accept suggestions.
- *Therapeutic Applications:* Ericksonian hypnosis and confusion techniques are effective for a wide range of therapeutic applications, including pain management, stress reduction, overcoming phobias, and behavior change.

Confusion and Ericksonian methods offer powerful, indirect ways to induce hypnosis, allowing the hypnotist to guide the subject into a trance without overt suggestion or formal induction techniques. By using cognitive disorientation, paradoxical statements, and subtle conversational patterns, the hypnotist can bypass the conscious mind's resistance and facilitate deep relaxation, therapeutic change, and improved suggestibility. These techniques are invaluable in a variety of settings, from therapeutic sessions to informal conversations, providing a versatile and effective means of hypnosis.

Chapter 10: Ethical Considerations

Understanding Ethics in Hypnosis

Hypnosis is a powerful tool with the potential to bring about profound changes in an individual's mind and behavior. However, with this power comes the responsibility of practicing hypnosis ethically and responsibly. Ethical considerations are vital in ensuring that hypnosis is used to help individuals in a respectful and beneficial manner while protecting their autonomy, dignity, and mental well-being.

In this chapter, we will explore the ethical responsibilities that hypnotists must adhere to when practicing hypnosis. This includes the guidelines for ensuring the safety, confidentiality, and consent of the subject, as well as respecting the boundaries of what hypnosis can and should be used for.

1. The Role of the Hypnotist

The hypnotist plays an important role as a facilitator of the subject's trance state. As with any professional relationship, the hypnotist has an ethical duty to act with integrity, respect, and care. This involves maintaining a supportive, non-coercive, and non-manipulative environment throughout the hypnotic process.

A key ethical principle is ensuring that hypnosis is used to benefit the subject, whether for therapeutic, personal development, or relaxation purposes. Hypnosis should never be used to harm, manipulate, or exploit a person's vulnerabilities.

Key Ethical Responsibilities of a Hypnotist:

- *Non-coercion:* The hypnotist must not use any form of force or coercion to induce hypnosis or make suggestions. All inductions and suggestions should be given in a respectful manner, with the subject's well-being in mind.

- *Respect for Autonomy*: The subject should always retain control over their thoughts and actions. Hypnosis should never be used to override a subject's personal will or values. The subject should have the ability to reject any suggestion at any time.
- *Trustworthiness*: Hypnotists must maintain trust with their clients, ensuring that any information revealed during hypnosis remains confidential and is handled appropriately.

2. Informed Consent

Informed consent is a fundamental ethical principle in any therapeutic or professional practice, and it is equally critical in hypnosis. Before beginning any hypnotic work, the hypnotist must obtain the subject's informed consent, which means that the subject fully understands what hypnosis entails, the potential risks and benefits, and their right to stop the process at any time. *Informed Consent Includes:*

- *Explanation of Hypnosis:* The hypnotist must explain what hypnosis is, how it works, and what to expect during the session. This helps demystify the process and reassures the subject that they will remain in control.
- *Clarification of Goals:* The hypnotist should discuss the goals of the session with the subject to ensure that both parties are aligned and that the subject's needs and desires are clearly understood.
- *Voluntary Participation:* It is essential that the subject voluntarily agrees to participate in the hypnosis session. Consent must be obtained without pressure or manipulation, ensuring that the subject feels free to decline or withdraw at any time.
- *Right to Withdraw:* The subject should be informed that they have the right to stop the hypnosis session at any point, and this decision will be respected by the hypnotist.

3. Confidentiality and Privacy

Confidentiality is another critical aspect of ethical hypnosis practice. A hypnotist is privy to potentially sensitive information disclosed by the subject during the session, especially in therapeutic contexts. This information must be kept private and confidential, unless the subject explicitly gives permission to share it.

Key Aspects of Confidentiality:

- *Safeguarding Information:* Hypnotists must ensure that any records, notes, or sessions are stored securely to prevent unauthorized access.
- *Limits of Confidentiality:* Hypnotists should explain the limits of confidentiality to their clients. There are some situations where confidentiality might need to be breached, such as when the subject is at risk of harm to themselves or others, but these exceptions must be clarified upfront.

4. Avoiding Manipulation and Exploitation

Hypnotists have a duty to avoid manipulating or exploiting their subjects. Hypnosis is a powerful state, and a subject may be more open to suggestions when in a trance. However, the hypnotist should never use this suggestibility for personal gain, to influence the subject's decisions, or to violate their personal beliefs and values.

Preventing Exploitation:

- *No Undue Influence:* Hypnotists should never use hypnosis to manipulate the subject's behavior, thoughts, or emotions for purposes that are not in the subject's best interest.
- *Respecting Boundaries:* Hypnotists should always respect the physical, emotional, and psychological boundaries of the subject. They should avoid engaging in any activities that could cause discomfort or harm to the subject, even if the subject appears willing or compliant.
- *Ethical Use of Hypnosis:* Hypnosis should never be used for trivial or frivolous purposes. For example, using hypnosis to persuade someone to make financial decisions, or to coerce them into actions against their will, is unethical and unacceptable.

5. Avoiding Harm and Psychological Risks

While hypnosis is generally safe, there are some risks involved, especially if performed improperly or inappropriately. Ethical hypnotists must be aware of potential risks and take steps to avoid causing harm.

Potential Psychological Risks:

- *Emotional Discomfort:* In some cases, deep emotional issues may arise during hypnosis, particularly in therapeutic settings. The hypnotist should be prepared to manage such emotions in a supportive manner and refer the subject to a qualified therapist if necessary.
- *False Memories:* Hypnosis, especially when used for age regression or memory retrieval, can sometimes lead to the creation of false memories. Hypnotists must be careful not to plant or suggest memories that were not actually experienced by the subject.
- *Overuse of Hypnosis:* Hypnosis should not be relied upon as the only tool for addressing a subject's issues. Overuse or dependence on hypnosis can create unrealistic expectations or prevent a person from seeking additional treatment or help when necessary.

6. Professional Competence and Training

Ethical hypnotists should only practice hypnosis if they have received proper training and certification. This ensures that they are competent in their practice and capable of addressing the needs of their subjects safely and effectively.

Ensuring Competence:

- *Continual Education:* Hypnotists should engage in ongoing education to stay up-to-date on the latest techniques and ethical guidelines in the field.
- *Certification and Licensing:* Depending on the region and the type of hypnosis being performed (e.g., therapeutic hypnosis), a hypnotist may be required to obtain specific certifications or licenses. Even if not required by law, certification is an important step to ensure competency and professionalism.
- *Referral to Other Professionals:* Hypnotists should recognize when a subject's issue requires the expertise of a licensed medical or

psychological professional, such as a therapist or doctor. In such cases, the hypnotist should refer the subject to the appropriate expert and avoid practicing outside their scope of competence.

Ethical considerations are paramount in the practice of hypnosis. Hypnotists must approach their work with respect for the autonomy, dignity, and well-being of their subjects. By adhering to the principles of informed consent, confidentiality, avoiding manipulation, and ensuring that their practice is competent and responsible, hypnotists can foster trust, safety, and effective outcomes for those they work with.

Ethical hypnosis not only protects the subjects but also ensures that the hypnotist can offer their services with integrity and professionalism, contributing to the overall growth and respect of the field of hypnosis.

When Not to Use Hypnosis: Knowing the Limitations and Risks Involved

While hypnosis is a powerful tool for facilitating therapeutic change, relaxation, and personal development, it is not appropriate for every situation or every individual. Hypnosis has limitations, and there are certain cases where its use could be harmful or ineffective. It's essential for hypnotists to be aware of these situations to avoid causing any psychological, emotional, or physical harm to their subjects.

In this section, we will explore the circumstances under which hypnosis should be avoided, highlighting the risks and ethical considerations that guide responsible practice.

1. Individuals with Severe Mental Health Disorders

Hypnosis should not be used with individuals who have severe mental health disorders such as schizophrenia, dissociative identity disorder (DID), or other serious psychotic conditions. These disorders may involve fragmented or impaired reality perception, making it difficult for the individual to fully distinguish between the hypnotic experience and reality.

Why Avoid Hypnosis in These Cases?

- *Risk of Disturbing Symptoms:* For individuals with severe mental health disorders, hypnosis may exacerbate symptoms such as delusions, paranoia, or dissociation. The hypnotic state could make it harder for these individuals to distinguish between their subconscious and external reality, potentially leading to confusion or distress.
- *Unpredictable Responses:* People with severe psychiatric disorders may have unpredictable responses to hypnosis, including resistance, dissociation, or emotional breakdowns during or after a session.

Alternative Approach:

Individuals with severe mental health conditions should seek treatment from licensed mental health professionals. In some cases, hypnosis might be integrated into their treatment plan under the supervision of a qualified therapist who specializes in both hypnosis and their specific condition.

2. Individuals Under the Influence of Drugs or Alcohol

Hypnosis should not be performed on individuals who are under the influence of drugs or alcohol. When someone is intoxicated or impaired, their cognitive functions, attention, and judgment are compromised, which can prevent them from entering a proper hypnotic state or make them more vulnerable to suggestion in an unhealthy way.

Why Avoid Hypnosis in These Cases?

- *Impaired Judgment and Suggestibility:* Under the influence of substances, a person's ability to make informed decisions or resist unwanted suggestions may be diminished. This could lead to unwanted or harmful outcomes, as the subject might be more suggestible and less able to exercise free will.
- *Risk of Misinterpretation:* The altered state caused by intoxication could interfere with the hypnotic process, potentially making the subject confused or unable to distinguish between the hypnosis and the effects of the substance they've consumed.

Alternative Approach:
Wait until the individual is sober and in a clear state of mind before attempting hypnosis. It is crucial that the person is able to understand the process and give informed consent.

3. People with Strong Resistance or Fear of Hypnosis

Hypnosis is not effective for people who have a strong resistance or fear of the process. If a person is unwilling or fearful, they may subconsciously block the induction process, making it difficult, if not impossible, to achieve a trance state.

Why Avoid Hypnosis in These Cases?

- *Inability to Enter Trance*: If someone has deep fears or significant skepticism about hypnosis, they may not be able to relax enough to enter a trance state, or they may resist the process altogether.
- *Increased Anxiety:* Attempting hypnosis on a person who is fearful may lead to heightened anxiety or distress rather than relaxation or therapeutic benefits. The person might feel pressured or uncomfortable, which could cause long-term negative associations with hypnosis.

Alternative Approach:
Instead of attempting hypnosis directly, the hypnotist should first work on addressing the fear or resistance through other methods such as education, relaxation techniques, or building trust. It may also help to clarify any misconceptions about hypnosis, addressing the fears by discussing what hypnosis actually involves.

4. When the Subject Has a History of Abuse or Trauma

Hypnosis can sometimes bring repressed memories or emotions to the surface, and for individuals who have experienced trauma or abuse, this can be overwhelming or even retraumatizing. Hypnosis may not always be suitable in these situations, especially if the subject has unresolved trauma that could be triggered by the process.

- *Risk of Re-traumatization:* For individuals with a history of trauma or abuse, hypnosis may unintentionally bring up painful or traumatic memories. Without proper therapeutic support, this could lead to emotional distress or re-traumatization.
- *Unresolved Emotional Issues:* If a person has unresolved emotional issues from past trauma, the hypnotic process could inadvertently cause confusion or emotional upheaval if the person is not adequately prepared to address those feelings.

Alternative Approach:

Hypnosis should only be used for individuals with a history of trauma or abuse under the guidance of a licensed therapist or counselor trained in trauma-informed care. The therapist may use hypnosis in conjunction with other therapeutic modalities to ensure the person feels safe and supported during the process.

5. During Certain Medical Conditions

Hypnosis should be approached with caution when used with individuals who have certain medical conditions, especially those with neurological disorders, epilepsy, or severe heart conditions. While hypnosis can sometimes be helpful in managing pain or stress, it should not replace medical treatment for serious health concerns.

Why Avoid Hypnosis in These Cases?

- *Potential for Unforeseen Reactions:* People with certain medical conditions may react unpredictably to hypnosis, particularly if their conditions involve the nervous system or cardiovascular system. For example, a person with epilepsy may experience seizures triggered by the relaxation or focused attention induced by hypnosis.
- *Not a Substitute for Medical Treatment:* Hypnosis should never be used as a substitute for medical diagnosis or treatment. In cases of serious illness or injury, medical professionals should be consulted,

and hypnosis can only be used as a complementary technique when cleared by the appropriate healthcare provider.

Alternative Approach:
Consult with the person's healthcare provider before attempting hypnosis. If hypnosis is appropriate, it should only be used in conjunction with other medical treatments and under professional supervision.

6. When the Hypnotist Lacks Proper Training or Experience

Hypnosis is a skill that requires knowledge, practice, and experience. It is crucial that hypnotists possess proper training, certification, and expertise before performing hypnosis, especially in sensitive or therapeutic situations. Practicing hypnosis without sufficient knowledge can be ineffective or even dangerous.

Why Avoid Hypnosis in These Cases?

- *Risk of Ineffective or Harmful Techniques:* Hypnosis performed by someone without adequate training may fail to achieve the desired results or, worse, cause harm to the subject. A poorly executed session could lead to confusion, emotional distress, or negative psychological effects.
- *Legal and Ethical Implications:* Performing hypnosis without the necessary qualifications or certification could expose the hypnotist to legal or ethical issues, especially in therapeutic contexts.

Alternative Approach:
Ensure that the hypnotist has received formal training from a reputable institution, is certified (where applicable), and has experience in the specific type of hypnosis being performed. Continuing education and professional development are essential for maintaining competence.

7. When It Conflicts with the Subject's Values or Beliefs

Hypnosis should never be used in a way that conflicts with a subject's deeply held values, beliefs, or personal boundaries. For example, if a person is against certain suggestions or if they have religious, cultural, or personal beliefs that conflict with the use of hypnosis, the hypnotist should refrain from using it. *Why Avoid Hypnosis in These Cases?*

- *Respect for Personal Beliefs:* Hypnosis should not be used to pressure someone into changing their beliefs, behaviors, or values, especially if doing so would be harmful to the individual's sense of self or well-being.
- *Potential for Ethical Violations*: Forcing or manipulating a subject to undergo hypnosis that contradicts their personal values could be seen as unethical and lead to feelings of betrayal or harm.

Alternative Approach:
Always discuss the subject's values and beliefs before starting hypnosis, and respect any boundaries they have. If hypnosis is not aligned with their beliefs or if they are uncomfortable, explore other methods that may be more suitable.

Know When to Say No

Hypnosis is a powerful tool, but it is not appropriate for every individual or every situation. As a responsible hypnotist, it is essential to recognize the limitations of hypnosis and avoid using it in cases where it may cause harm or be ineffective. Knowing when **not** to use hypnosis is just as important as knowing how to use it effectively.

By recognizing the risks and ethical considerations involved in hypnosis, and respecting the autonomy and well-being of the subject, the hypnotist can practice responsibly and with integrity, ensuring that hypnosis is only used in situations where it can bring real benefit to the individual.

Professional Boundaries and Consent: Respecting the Subject's Autonomy and Consent During Hypnosis

In any professional relationship, maintaining clear boundaries and ensuring informed consent are essential to ensuring the safety and well-being of the subject. This is especially true in hypnosis, where the hypnotist has access to the subject's mind in a vulnerable state. The hypnotist must respect the subject's autonomy, preferences, and personal boundaries at all times, fostering an environment of trust, safety, and respect.

This section will explore the importance of professional boundaries in hypnosis and the ethical requirements for obtaining and maintaining consent throughout the hypnotic process.

1. Understanding Professional Boundaries

Professional boundaries refer to the clear, ethical lines between the hypnotist and the subject, designed to protect both parties and preserve the integrity of the hypnotic relationship. Boundaries ensure that the hypnotist maintains a professional demeanor, refrains from overstepping their role, and ensures the safety and comfort of the subject at all times.

Key Aspects of Professional Boundaries:

- *Respectful Behavior:* The hypnotist should always maintain professionalism, using respectful language and behavior in all interactions. Any form of inappropriate conduct, whether verbal or non-verbal, is unacceptable and can damage the trust required for effective hypnosis.
- *Emotional Distance:* While it's important for the hypnotist to build rapport and trust, it's equally important to maintain an appropriate emotional distance. The hypnotist should not become overly involved in the subject's personal life or create an emotional dependency on the hypnosis sessions.
- *Avoiding Dual Relationships:* Hypnotists should avoid dual relationships, where they have both a professional and personal connection with the subject. This could lead to conflicts of interest, compromised objectivity, and blurred boundaries.
- *Maintaining a Safe Physical Space:* The hypnotist should always ensure that the physical environment in which hypnosis is conducted is safe, comfortable, and private. This helps ensure the subject feels physically and emotionally secure.

2. Informed Consent: The Foundation of Hypnosis

Informed consent is a core ethical principle in hypnosis and refers to the subject's right to fully understand what hypnosis entails, the goals of the session, the potential benefits and risks, and their ability to withdraw consent at any time.

Informed consent is a *continuous* process, not just a one-time agreement. Consent must be revisited throughout the hypnotic experience to ensure that the subject feels in control and empowered.

Steps for Obtaining Informed Consent:

- *Clear Explanation:* The hypnotist must provide the subject with a clear explanation of what hypnosis is, how it works, and what to expect during the session. This includes explaining that hypnosis is a natural state and that the subject will retain control throughout the process.

- *Discussing Goals and Expectations:* The hypnotist should work with the subject to establish the goals of the session. The subject should be able to ask questions about the process and have their concerns addressed before agreeing to proceed.

- *Explaining Risks and Benefits*: The hypnotist should explain both the potential benefits and any risks associated with hypnosis. For example, hypnosis may help with relaxation, stress relief, or habit change, but there may also be emotional reactions or discomfort when addressing sensitive topics.

- *Voluntary Participation:* The subject must agree to participate voluntarily, without any form of pressure or coercion. They must also understand that they are free to stop the session at any time.

- *Right to Withdraw*: The subject should be made aware that they can withdraw consent at any point during the session, and that this decision will be respected. This ensures that the subject does not feel trapped or manipulated in any way.

Documenting Consent: In many cases, it's a good practice for the hypnotist to have the subject sign a consent form, especially in professional settings like therapy. This document serves as evidence that the subject understands and agrees to the process.

3. Respecting Autonomy During Hypnosis

Autonomy refers to the subject's right to make their own decisions, and it is a crucial aspect of any hypnotic session. A subject's autonomy must be respected at all times, both before and during the session.

Key Aspects of Respecting Autonomy:

- *Control Over the Session:* Throughout the hypnosis session, the subject must always feel in control of their experience. While they may relax deeply and follow the hypnotist's suggestions, they retain the ability to accept or reject any suggestion at any time.
- *Avoiding Coercion*: Hypnosis should never be used as a tool for manipulation or coercion. The hypnotist must refrain from giving suggestions that are against the subject's best interests, values, or personal beliefs.
- *Clear Boundaries for Suggestions*: The hypnotist should avoid suggestions that could push the subject to do something they would never do consciously, such as revealing deeply personal information or engaging in activities that go against their moral or ethical beliefs.
- *Empowering the Subject:* The hypnotist should always empower the subject, allowing them to feel confident in their ability to make decisions during the session. The hypnotist's role is to guide and support the subject, not to control or dominate their actions.

4. Ongoing Consent Throughout the Process

Consent is not a one-time agreement; it is an ongoing process that continues throughout the session. A subject may change their mind, feel uncomfortable, or become hesitant at any point, and the hypnotist must be prepared to respect their wishes and adjust accordingly.

Regular Check-Ins:

Throughout the hypnosis session, it's important for the hypnotist to periodically check in with the subject to ensure that they remain comfortable and willing to proceed. This can be done by asking simple, non-intrusive questions like:

- "How are you feeling right now?"
- "Is there anything you would like to adjust or stop?"
- "Do you feel comfortable continuing?"

Recognizing Discomfort:

If the subject shows any signs of discomfort, resistance, or distress, the hypnotist must respect their boundaries and take immediate action to address the situation. This may involve guiding the subject out of the hypnotic state, offering reassurance, or halting the session if needed.

5. Confidentiality and Privacy

In addition to respecting autonomy and consent, maintaining confidentiality is an essential part of creating a trusting relationship with the subject. The hypnotist should ensure that any personal information disclosed during the session remains private, unless there is explicit permission to share it, or if there is a legal obligation to report it.

Key Principles of Confidentiality:

- *Secure Handling of Information:* Any information gathered during the session should be treated with the utmost care. This includes both verbal disclosures and any records kept by the hypnotist (e.g., session notes).
- *Limitations of Confidentiality:* The hypnotist should inform the subject of any limits to confidentiality, such as legal requirements to report information in cases of imminent harm, abuse, or threats to safety.
- *Ensuring Privacy:* The hypnotist must provide a private and secure environment for the session, ensuring that no one else can overhear or interrupt the conversation. Privacy helps the subject feel safe and supported throughout the process.

6. When Boundaries Are Crossed

In some cases, a subject may feel that their boundaries have been crossed, either intentionally or unintentionally. The hypnotist must be sensitive to any signs of discomfort, and if boundaries are violated, they must take immediate action to correct the situation and prevent it from happening in the future.

Signs of Boundary Violation:

- *Physical Discomfort:* The subject may feel physically uncomfortable, either due to the hypnotist's actions or the setting.
- *Emotional Distress:* The subject may express feelings of distress, confusion, or anxiety during or after the session.
- *Resistance or Withdrawal:* The subject may start resisting suggestions or display signs of withdrawal, such as disengaging from the process or becoming defensive.

If a subject expresses discomfort, the hypnotist should stop the session and ask for clarification on what went wrong. The hypnotist should also apologize if necessary, reassure the subject, and make changes to ensure that the boundaries are respected in future sessions.

The Importance of Respectful Practice

Respecting professional boundaries and ensuring ongoing consent are cornerstones of ethical hypnosis practice. Hypnosis is an intimate and vulnerable process, and it is crucial that the hypnotist fosters an environment of trust, safety, and respect throughout the session. By maintaining clear boundaries, empowering the subject, and regularly checking in for consent, the hypnotist ensures a positive and effective experience.

Through ethical conduct, hypnosis can be a powerful tool for personal growth, relaxation, and healing, while always safeguarding the subject's autonomy, dignity, and well-being.

Chapter 11: Self-Improvement for the Hypnotist

Developing Your Skills: Exercises and Techniques to Improve Your Hypnosis Skills
As a hypnotist, continuous self-improvement is crucial for both your own growth and your ability to help others effectively. Mastery in hypnosis is not simply about learning specific techniques but also about developing your ability to read people, communicate effectively, and adapt to each individual. This chapter offers exercises and strategies that can help you refine your skills, increase your confidence, and become a more effective hypnotist.

1. Practice Active Listening and Observation

Exercise: Active Listening Practice
Effective hypnosis starts with being able to listen attentively to your subjects. This means not only hearing their words but also understanding their feelings, body language, and underlying emotions.

- *How to Practice:* Pair up with a friend or colleague and engage in a conversation where one person speaks and the other practices active listening. The listener should focus on:
    - *Verbal Cues*: Pay attention to the tone, pace, and words the person uses.
    - *Non-verbal Cues:* Notice body language, facial expressions, and gestures.
    - *Empathy and Reflection:* Respond with empathy, and reflect back what you hear to ensure you understand the emotions and ideas behind the words.

Why It's Important:

Listening carefully helps you tailor your hypnosis sessions to the unique needs and concerns of each individual. It also allows you to spot resistance or discomfort, which is essential for adapting your approach and building trust.

2. Develop Your Rapport-Building Skills
Exercise: Rapport Building with Mirror Technique
Establishing rapport is a fundamental part of any hypnosis session. Practicing rapport-building techniques outside of formal hypnosis sessions can help you become more intuitive in forming connections.

- *How to Practice:* Engage in casual conversation with someone and subtly mirror their posture, gestures, and tone of voice. This should be done naturally—avoid overdoing it or making the mirroring too obvious.
    - *Step 1:* Mirror body language—if they lean forward, lean forward too.
    - *Step 2:* Match their tone and pace of speech—if they speak slowly and softly, mirror that rhythm.
    - *Step 3:* Use similar phrasing or words to build connection.

Why It's Important:
Rapport is essential for creating a comfortable environment where the subject feels safe and understood. By practicing mirroring, you will be better equipped to build trust quickly and guide subjects into a deep, relaxed state.

3. Develop Your Language Skills for Hypnotic Suggestions
Exercise: Creating Hypnotic Language Patterns
Language is one of the most powerful tools you have as a hypnotist. The ability to use language to guide, direct, and influence your subject's thoughts is critical. This exercise helps you develop the specific language patterns needed to craft effective hypnotic suggestions.

- *How to Practice:* Write down a few simple suggestions that can be used in various contexts (e.g., for relaxation, confidence, stress relief). Then, practice transforming them into hypnotic language patterns. Here are some ways to do so:
    - *Indirect Suggestions:* Instead of giving direct commands, use subtle phrasing like, "You may begin to notice..." or "It's possible that you'll find

it easy to..."

- ○ *Embedded Commands:* Learn to hide commands within longer sentences. For example: "As you sit back and relax, you might find yourself feeling deeply at ease."
- ○ *Future Pacing:* Practice using suggestions that imagine a future event. "In the coming days, you'll notice how much more relaxed you are each time you face a challenge."

Why It's Important:

Learning to speak in a hypnotic, suggestive way helps you better influence and guide your subjects. The ability to use subtle, indirect language will also make your suggestions feel more natural and less imposing.

4. Hone Your Ability to Read and Adapt to Subjects

Exercise: Emotional Awareness Practice

Being able to pick up on emotional cues from your subjects is essential for understanding their responses and adjusting your technique accordingly. This exercise will help you sharpen your ability to read emotions, both verbal and non-verbal.

- • *How to Practice:* Engage in conversations with people who may be in different emotional states (e.g., happy, frustrated, anxious, relaxed). Focus on:
  - ○ *Non-verbal Cues:* Pay close attention to their body language, posture, and facial expressions.
  - ○ *Verbal Cues:* Notice the tone and speed of their speech, as well as any changes in their voice.
  - ○ *Emotional States:* Try to identify the emotional state they are in without them explicitly telling you.

Why It's Important:

Being emotionally attuned to your subject allows you to tailor your hypnosis approach. If you sense discomfort, resistance, or anxiety, you can adjust your technique to ensure the session remains smooth and beneficial. This skill is also important for pacing, where you learn to go slower or faster depending on the subject's comfort level.

5. Strengthen Your Self-Confidence and Focus

Exercise: Self-Hypnosis for Confidence

Confidence is a cornerstone of effective hypnosis. If you are not confident in your ability to guide someone into a trance or suggest changes, your subject may pick up on this and feel less relaxed. This exercise helps boost your confidence and allows you to manage any nervousness you may experience.

- *How to Practice:* Use self-hypnosis to help you relax and focus before sessions. Create a simple self-hypnosis script where you reinforce your own confidence:
    - Induce a state of relaxation with deep breathing or progressive muscle relaxation.
    - Use positive affirmations: "I am a skilled and confident hypnotist. I trust my abilities to guide my subjects."
    - Visualize successful hypnosis sessions and imagine your subjects responding positively to your suggestions.

Why It's Important:

Self-confidence enhances your ability to be a calming, authoritative presence for your subjects. If you can manage your own anxiety or self-doubt, you will be more focused and effective during sessions, which leads to better results.

6. Expand Your Knowledge of Advanced Hypnotic Techniques

Exercise: Study and Practice Ericksonian Methods

As you advance in your hypnosis journey, you'll want to explore more sophisticated techniques, such as those developed by Milton Erickson. These include indirect suggestion, conversational hypnosis, and metaphorical storytelling.

- *How to Practice:* Read books or articles on Ericksonian hypnosis. Then, practice integrating these techniques into your own sessions. For instance:
    - Use metaphors and stories to bypass resistance and communicate with the subconscious mind.
    - Practice permissive suggestions, where you present ideas gently, allowing the subject to feel they are in control.

- Experiment with open-ended questions that guide the subject toward their own insights (e.g., "What do you think might happen if you imagined yourself in a peaceful place?").

Why It's Important:

Ericksonian techniques offer powerful methods for creating deeper, more effective hypnosis experiences. By mastering these advanced techniques, you can enhance your flexibility and ability to work with a wide variety of subjects and issues.

7. Continuous Learning and Feedback

Exercise: Record and Review Your Sessions

To ensure continuous improvement, recording your hypnosis sessions and reviewing them afterward is an excellent way to refine your approach. It allows you to analyze your techniques and make adjustments.

- *How to Practice:* With the consent of your subjects, record your hypnosis sessions. Afterward, listen carefully to the language you used, the pacing, and the tone of your voice. Reflect on areas that went well and those that could be improved.
  - Pay attention to any resistance or challenges that arose during the session.
  - Assess whether your language was clear, your rapport was strong, and your techniques were effective.

Why It's Important:

Self-reflection and feedback are vital for any hypnotist striving for mastery. By analyzing your own work, you'll identify areas for improvement and gain greater insight into how to handle different subjects and situations.

Lifelong Learning for Hypnotists

Developing as a hypnotist is a continuous journey. By practicing these exercises, improving your listening skills, refining your language, building rapport, and gaining experience, you'll enhance both your technical abilities and your intuitive understanding of hypnosis. The more you practice, the more confident and effective you will become, enabling you to help your subjects achieve deeper transformations and greater success. Remember, hypnosis is not just about learning specific techniques—it's about growing as a communicator, a listener, and a guide. Keep honing your skills and always be open to learning.

Overcoming Personal Blocks: How to Overcome Your Own Limiting Beliefs as a Practitioner

As a hypnotist, your effectiveness is not only dependent on the techniques you use but also on your mindset and personal belief systems. Like any skill, hypnosis requires confidence, self-belief, and emotional resilience. Unfortunately, personal blocks such as self-doubt, fear of failure, or limiting beliefs can significantly hinder your ability to perform effectively and confidently. This section will focus on how to identify and overcome these internal barriers so that you can become a more skilled, effective, and confident practitioner.

1. Identifying Limiting Beliefs

Before you can overcome limiting beliefs, it is crucial to first identify them. These are negative thought patterns or doubts that can undermine your confidence and prevent you from progressing.

Common Limiting Beliefs for Hypnotists:

- "I'm not good enough to help others." This belief might arise from a lack of experience or a fear of making mistakes.
- "I can't hypnotize everyone." This may be rooted in doubts about your abilities or fears of failure if a subject doesn't respond.
- "I need more training before I can be effective." Constantly feeling unprepared or like you need more knowledge can delay progress.
- "Hypnosis doesn't work on certain people." This limiting belief can come from a fear that some people might not be receptive to hypnosis.

How to Identify Them:

- *Self-Reflection:* Take some time to reflect on your thoughts and emotions around hypnosis. Are there any recurring negative patterns? Do you feel anxious or doubtful before performing hypnosis on others?
- *Feedback from Others:* Sometimes, the feedback you receive can highlight your insecurities. If a subject responds negatively or if you feel unsure about a session's success, it may reinforce your limiting beliefs.
- *Journaling:* Write about your experiences with hypnosis. Often, seeing your thoughts on paper can help you uncover patterns of self-doubt and fear.

2. Reframing Negative Beliefs

Once you've identified your limiting beliefs, the next step is to reframe them into more positive, empowering thoughts. This involves challenging the belief and replacing it with a more constructive perspective.

Techniques for Reframing:

- *Cognitive Behavioral Therapy (CBT) Techniques:* CBT focuses on identifying negative thoughts and replacing them with more positive ones. For example:
    - Negative Thought: "I'm not good enough to hypnotize people."
    - Reframed Thought: "I am continuously learning and improving my skills. Every session helps me become a better hypnotist."
- *Affirmations*: Use positive affirmations to reinforce your ability and self-worth. For example, say to yourself: "I am skilled at guiding people into a hypnotic state. I am confident and capable."
- *Visualizing Success:* Imagine yourself succeeding in hypnosis sessions, seeing your subjects respond positively and experiencing successful outcomes. Visualization builds self-confidence and rewires your brain to believe in your capabilities.

3. Confronting Fear of Failure

Fear of failure is a major block for many practitioners, especially when starting out. You might worry that you will not be able to hypnotize someone successfully or that they won't respond. This fear can create anxiety, making you less effective.

How to Overcome It:

- *Start Small:* Begin with simple, low-pressure sessions. Practice hypnosis with friends or family who are supportive and understanding. This will help you gain experience without the fear of failure.
- *Shift Your Perspective on Failure:* Reframe failure as an opportunity to learn rather than a setback. Every experience—whether successful or not—provides valuable insight into how you can improve. Remember that even experienced practitioners occasionally face setbacks.
- *Create a Supportive Environment:* Surround yourself with others who are also learning or practicing hypnosis. Sharing experiences and discussing challenges can help alleviate your fears and reinforce the idea that failure is a part of the learning process.

4. Building Confidence Through Experience

Confidence grows with experience. The more you practice hypnosis, the more confident you will become in your abilities. However, gaining that confidence requires consistent effort and stepping outside your comfort zone.

How to Build Confidence:

- *Practice Regularly:* Make hypnosis a regular part of your life. Practice self-hypnosis, work with volunteers, or practice techniques with fellow hypnotists. The more you practice, the more natural it will feel.
- *Track Progress:* Keep track of your successes, even the small ones. Whether it's a subject going into light trance or an improvement in their issue after hypnosis, noting your progress will boost your confidence over time.
- *Celebrate Small Wins:* Each successful session, no matter how small, is

a step toward greater proficiency. Celebrate these wins to reinforce your belief in your abilities.

5. Overcoming Imposter Syndrome

Imposter syndrome is the feeling that you are a "fraud" or that you don't deserve your successes, despite evidence to the contrary. Many new practitioners experience this, believing that they don't have the right to help others or that they are unqualified.

How to Overcome Imposter Syndrome:

- *Acknowledge Your Growth:* Reflect on how far you've come. You are constantly learning, and every step forward means you are improving.
- *Seek Support:* Reach out to mentors or fellow practitioners for support and guidance. Talking to others in the field can help you realize that even experienced hypnotists faced similar feelings when they were starting out.
- *Focus on the Benefits You Offer:* Remember that hypnosis is a tool that can help people achieve their goals, improve their well-being, and overcome challenges. Your ability to provide this service is valuable, regardless of your experience level.

6. Cultivating a Growth Mindset

A growth mindset is the belief that abilities and intelligence can be developed over time through effort and perseverance. This mindset is essential for overcoming limiting beliefs and improving as a hypnotist.

How to Develop a Growth Mindset:

- *Embrace Challenges:* See challenges as opportunities to grow rather than obstacles. If a subject doesn't respond well to a session, view it as a chance to refine your techniques.
- *Be Open to Feedback:* Accept constructive feedback from others, whether it's from clients, mentors, or peers. Feedback helps you identify areas where you can improve and enhances your learning process.

- *Focus on Learning, Not Perfection:* Understand that no one is perfect, and you do not need to be perfect either. Focus on learning, improving, and growing, rather than achieving flawless results from the outset.

7. Strengthening Your Mindset for Success

Hypnosis is as much about mental strength as it is about technique. As a hypnotist, your ability to manage your own thoughts and emotions can significantly impact your practice. By cultivating mental clarity and emotional resilience, you can overcome your personal blocks and become a more successful practitioner.

How to Strengthen Your Mindset:

- *Mindfulness Practices*: Incorporate mindfulness techniques such as meditation, breathing exercises, or yoga into your routine. These practices help you clear mental clutter, reduce stress, and stay focused during hypnosis sessions.
- *Visualization of Success:* Regularly visualize yourself confidently guiding subjects into hypnosis and successfully achieving positive outcomes. This visualization creates a mental roadmap for success and reinforces the belief that you are capable.
- *Self-Compassion:* Be kind to yourself. Recognize that all practitioners, even experienced ones, face challenges and setbacks. Be patient with your own growth and acknowledge your efforts along the way.

Overcoming Blocks for Long-Term Success

As a hypnotist, you will encounter challenges, both external and internal. Overcoming your personal limiting beliefs, building confidence, and embracing a growth mindset are key to long-term success. By addressing your mental and emotional barriers, you can become a more effective, confident, and empowered practitioner. Remember that your journey toward mastery in hypnosis is ongoing, and overcoming your personal blocks is a crucial part of that journey. Stay patient with yourself, practice consistently, and focus on continuous learning and growth.

Embrace Lifelong Learning

Becoming a highly skilled and effective hypnotist requires an ongoing commitment to learning. By exploring books, taking courses, attending conferences, and working with mentors, you can continue to evolve as a practitioner. Hypnosis is a field that requires both technical expertise and emotional intelligence, so honing your skills in both areas will help you become a more competent and confident practitioner. With dedication to continual learning and self-reflection, you can master hypnosis and make a lasting impact in your practice.

Chapter 12: Troubleshooting and Problem Solving: Dealing with Difficult Subjects; When Hypnosis Doesn't Work; Recognizing and Addressing Negative Reactions

How to Handle Subjects Who Are Resistant or Difficult to Hypnotize
In hypnosis practice, encountering resistance or difficulty in hypnotizing a subject is not uncommon. Whether it's due to skepticism, fear, or an inability to relax fully, certain individuals may present challenges during the induction process. Understanding why a subject might be difficult to hypnotize and learning strategies to overcome these obstacles is crucial for any hypnotist's success.

1. Understanding Resistance in Hypnosis

Resistance during hypnosis can manifest in several ways, such as:

- *Skepticism*: Some subjects may not believe in the effectiveness of hypnosis or may doubt their ability to enter a trance. This can create a mental block that makes induction more difficult.
- *Fear or Anxiety:* Fear of losing control or of being unable to "wake up" can cause the subject to resist the process unconsciously.
- *Overactive Mind:* Individuals with racing thoughts or a constant stream of mental activity may struggle to relax and focus enough for hypnosis to work.
- *Inability to Let Go:* Some people may have trouble relinquishing control and allowing themselves to be guided into a trance state.
- *Physical Discomfort:* If a subject is physically uncomfortable or in pain, it may be hard for them to focus on relaxation or deepening

techniques.

By understanding these sources of resistance, a hypnotist can take the right steps to address them and increase the chances of a successful session.

2. Strategies for Handling Resistance
Building Rapport and Trust
Building a strong rapport is essential for any hypnosis session. A resistant subject is more likely to relax if they feel they are in a safe and trusting environment. Take extra time to connect with your subject and make them feel comfortable before attempting to hypnotize them.

- *Start with Casual Conversation:* Before beginning the hypnosis process, talk to your subject in a relaxed, non-authoritative manner. This helps ease any tension and sets a comfortable tone.
- *Explain the Process:* Clearly describe what hypnosis is and what they can expect during the session. Make sure to address any misconceptions they may have (e.g., the fear of "losing control") and reassure them that they will remain in control at all times.
- *Gauge Their Comfort Level:* Pay attention to body language and verbal cues. If your subject seems uneasy or uncomfortable, pause and address their concerns.

Adjusting Your Approach
Not everyone responds to hypnosis in the same way, so it's important to be adaptable in your approach.

- *Modify Induction Techniques:* If a subject isn't responding to one induction method, switch to another. For example, if they're struggling with progressive relaxation, try an eye fixation or guided visualization technique.
- *Use a Softer, Calmer Voice:* For subjects who are anxious or tense, adjust the tone of your voice to be slower, softer, and more soothing. This can help them relax and become more receptive.

- *Use Simple Language*: If a subject is highly analytical or overthinking, simplify your language to ensure they can focus on the process instead of trying to figure out how it works.

Addressing Fear and Anxiety

Fear or anxiety about the hypnosis process is one of the most common barriers to a successful session. Many people are afraid of being "out of control" or "stuck in hypnosis."

- *Reassure the Subject:* Make sure they know that they will always be in control and that they can come out of the hypnotic state at any time if they wish. Explain that hypnosis is a natural state of focused attention and relaxation.
- *Start with a Relaxing Pre-Induction:* Before formally attempting to induce hypnosis, guide the subject through a brief relaxation exercise. This could include deep breathing or progressive muscle relaxation to help reduce tension and anxiety.
- *Offer a Safe Word:* If the subject is particularly nervous, you can introduce a "safe word" that they can say if they feel uncomfortable or want to stop the session. This gives them a sense of control and security.

3. Techniques for Difficult-to-Hypnotize Individuals

Some subjects may be more resistant to hypnosis than others. This can be due to a variety of factors, including skepticism or an inability to relax. Here are several techniques to help overcome resistance in these individuals:

Utilize Direct and Indirect Suggestions

Some subjects may respond better to direct commands, while others may be more responsive to indirect, conversational suggestions.

- *Direct Suggestions:* Direct suggestions involve clear, straightforward instructions, such as "You will now begin to relax deeply." These can be effective for people who respond well to authority or clear guidance.

- *Indirect Suggestions:* These suggestions are more subtle and can be phrased as metaphors or stories. For example, "Imagine that your body is like a heavy stone sinking gently into a calm sea." These types of suggestions are often more effective for creative or resistant subjects.

Try Rapid or Instant Inductions

For subjects who are highly resistant or skeptical, rapid inductions can sometimes be more effective than traditional progressive relaxation techniques. Rapid inductions involve creating a sudden shift in the subject's focus or attention, making it easier to bypass mental resistance.

- *Handshake Induction*: A common rapid induction where the hypnotist offers their hand for a handshake, then suddenly guides the subject's hand downward, catching them off guard and inducing a trance.
- *Shock Induction:* This involves a sudden, unexpected action, such as a loud clap or verbal command, that interrupts the subject's thought process and helps them relax immediately.

Use the Reframing Technique

For subjects who resist hypnosis because they fear it will not work or believe they are "immune," the reframing technique can help. This technique involves changing the way the subject perceives hypnosis. For example, if they believe they cannot be hypnotized, you can say:

- "Some people believe they can't be hypnotized because they think they need to be more relaxed or focused. But the truth is, anyone can enter a hypnotic state because it's simply a state of heightened awareness, not a deep sleep or unconsciousness."

This change in perspective can help reduce resistance by transforming their skepticism into curiosity.

4. Encouraging Relaxation and Focus

Some subjects may have trouble relaxing enough to enter a trance. For these individuals, you may need to encourage relaxation more intensely.

- *Use Guided Relaxation:* If your subject has trouble relaxing, guide them through a detailed relaxation process, focusing on each part of the body. For example, "Relax your forehead, let go of any tension in your face, feel your eyelids grow heavier..."
- *Focus on Breathing:* Encourage slow, deep breathing, as focusing on the breath can help ease tension and improve focus. Guide them to take deep, rhythmic breaths, and assure them that relaxation will happen gradually.
- *Create a Calm Environment:* Ensure the room is quiet, dimly lit, and free of distractions. Sometimes, external stimuli can make it more difficult for a subject to relax.

5. Working with Analytical or Logical Minds

Some subjects, especially those who are very logical or analytical, may overthink the process and have difficulty allowing themselves to enter a trance. These individuals tend to question every step, which can interfere with relaxation and the induction process.

- *Encourage a "Letting Go" Mentality:* Gently remind them that hypnosis is not about control but about allowing themselves to relax and let go of the need to analyze everything.
- *Use a Logical Approach*: For analytical types, try framing hypnosis as a process of focusing attention rather than "losing control." Explain that the more they relax and focus, the more likely they are to enter a trance.
- *Gradual Induction*: Rather than trying to induce a deep trance immediately, consider using a more gradual approach that allows them to ease into hypnosis step-by-step.

6. When to Stop and Try Again Later

Sometimes, despite your best efforts, a subject may not be ready or willing to undergo hypnosis in that session. It's important to know when to stop and give them space to process the experience before attempting again.

- *Avoid Pressuring the Subject:* If a subject is showing clear resistance or discomfort, it's important to stop the session and explain that it's okay. Pushing too hard can cause the person to become more resistant and increase anxiety.
- *Suggest Future Sessions:* If the subject is willing, suggest trying hypnosis again at a later time, as they may need more time to relax or build trust in the process.

Dealing with difficult or resistant subjects is a natural part of any hypnotist's journey. The key to success lies in being adaptable, understanding the reasons behind resistance, and using appropriate techniques to help the subject relax and focus. By building rapport, adjusting your methods, and applying patience and flexibility, you can increase your chances of success even with the most challenging subjects. Every difficult session is an opportunity to learn and refine your skills, so embrace these challenges as part of your growth as a hypnotist.

When Hypnosis Doesn't Work

Understanding Why Hypnosis May Not Be Effective in Some Cases

While hypnosis is a powerful tool for many individuals, there are times when it may not be effective. Understanding why hypnosis may fail or be less effective in certain cases can help the hypnotist adjust their approach, manage expectations, and ensure that both the subject and practitioner remain confident in the process.

1. Lack of Willingness or Desire

One of the most fundamental factors in the success of hypnosis is the subject's willingness and desire to be hypnotized. If a person is not genuinely open to the process or does not believe in its effectiveness, it can significantly reduce the chances of a successful session.

- *Skepticism*: Some people may enter a session with doubts about hypnosis, viewing it as pseudoscience or trickery. This skepticism can create mental resistance, making it difficult for them to relax and enter a hypnotic state.

- *Lack of Desire:* Even if a subject does not actively resist, if they are not motivated to change or achieve a specific goal (e.g., quitting smoking, managing stress), the effectiveness of hypnosis will likely be diminished.

Solution: To increase effectiveness, address any concerns or misconceptions before starting the session. Establishing clear goals and ensuring that the subject truly wants to experience change will improve the chances of success.

2. Inadequate Rapport and Trust

Hypnosis relies heavily on the relationship between the hypnotist and the subject. If trust and rapport have not been properly established, it can hinder the subject's ability to relax and respond to suggestions.

- *Lack of Connection*: If the subject does not feel comfortable or does not trust the hypnotist, they may resist entering a trance. This lack of connection can manifest as physical tension, nervousness, or a distracted state of mind.
- *Miscommunication:* If the subject does not feel understood or is uncomfortable with the way the hypnotist communicates, it may prevent them from fully engaging in the process.

Solution: Spend time building rapport with the subject before starting hypnosis. Create a relaxed and open environment, explain the process clearly, and ensure that the subject feels comfortable and heard.

3. Fear and Anxiety

Fear and anxiety are common barriers to successful hypnosis. A subject who is afraid of losing control or has misconceptions about the process may resist the trance state, either consciously or unconsciously.

- *Fear of Losing Control:* Some subjects fear that they may not be able to "wake up" or regain control of their actions during hypnosis, which can prevent them from fully surrendering to the process.

- *General Anxiety*: High levels of anxiety, especially in subjects with generalized anxiety disorder, can make it difficult for them to relax enough to enter a trance.

Solution: Address these fears upfront by reassuring the subject that they will always be in control. Take extra time to explain that hypnosis is a natural, safe, and relaxed state of heightened awareness, and that they can always "snap out" of it if they need to. Consider using relaxation techniques or guided imagery to reduce anxiety before attempting hypnosis.

4. Analytical or Overactive Minds

People with highly analytical or overactive minds may find it challenging to relax and focus their attention. These individuals tend to overthink and may struggle to quiet their mental chatter, which is necessary for hypnosis to be effective.

- *Difficulty Letting Go:* Analytical types may attempt to analyze every step of the process or question whether they are doing it "correctly." This can prevent them from allowing themselves to enter a relaxed, suggestible state.
- *Hyperactivity*: Individuals with an overactive mind may find it hard to slow their thoughts, making deep relaxation and concentration difficult to achieve.

Solution: For these individuals, it may help to use techniques such as conversational hypnosis, or indirect suggestions to bypass the critical mind. A more structured or logical approach, such as progressive relaxation or counting, may also help them ease into the process more comfortably.

5. Physical Discomfort or Exhaustion

Physical discomfort, pain, or extreme exhaustion can also interfere with hypnosis. If a subject is in pain, too tired, or physically uncomfortable, they may be unable to relax fully or focus their attention, making it difficult to enter a trance.

- *Pain or Illness:* Chronic pain or illness can create distractions that prevent a subject from entering a deep state of relaxation.

- *Lack of Rest*: If the subject is overly fatigued or has not had enough sleep, their energy levels may be too low to engage effectively in the hypnosis process.

Solution: Ensure that the subject is in a comfortable environment. Consider addressing any physical discomfort before proceeding with hypnosis (e.g., offering a cushion or blanket, adjusting room temperature, etc.). For tired subjects, it may be better to schedule the session at a time when they feel more rested and energized.

6. Inappropriate Expectations

Sometimes, hypnosis fails because the subject's expectations are unrealistic. For example, a person may expect an immediate, dramatic change after just one session, or they may expect to be "completely cured" of a complex issue without sustained effort.

- *Unrealistic Goals:* If the subject expects instant results, they may become frustrated or discouraged if they don't experience rapid improvement.
- *Misunderstanding of Hypnosis:* People may have misconceptions about what hypnosis can do (e.g., the belief that hypnosis can make someone stop smoking after one session or that it can solve deep-seated psychological issues instantly).

Solution: Ensure that expectations are properly managed before the session begins. Explain that hypnosis is a tool for facilitating change, but that results may take time and require multiple sessions. Focus on the process rather than immediate outcomes.

7. Mental Health Conditions and Psychiatric Disorders

In some cases, hypnosis may not be effective if the subject has certain mental health conditions or psychiatric disorders that require specialized treatment. Conditions like severe depression, schizophrenia, or dissociative disorders may complicate the hypnosis process.

- *Severe Psychological Issues:* People with severe psychological or emotional disturbances may find it difficult to relax or accept suggestions. They may also experience negative reactions to hypnosis.

- *Incompatible Therapy:* Some mental health conditions may require a different therapeutic approach, and hypnosis may not be the most appropriate tool for addressing the issue at hand.

Solution: Before conducting hypnosis, always assess whether the person has any psychological conditions that may make hypnosis unsuitable. If in doubt, refer the subject to a licensed mental health professional. Hypnosis should never be used as a substitute for appropriate mental health care, especially in severe cases.

8. Inability to Achieve a Deep State of Trance

Not everyone is equally susceptible to hypnosis. Some individuals are highly responsive and can enter a deep trance quickly, while others may only experience light or shallow trances. While this does not mean that hypnosis has failed, it can impact the depth of work that can be done.

- *Shallow Trance:* Some subjects may experience only a light state of hypnosis, which may limit the effectiveness of certain therapeutic techniques. In these cases, suggestions may not have the same impact.
- *Resistance to Deep Trance*: Some individuals may have difficulty relaxing deeply enough to reach a state where therapeutic work, such as regression or deep suggestions, is possible.

Solution: Focus on working with the depth of trance that the subject achieves. Even if they are not deeply hypnotized, you can still use light trance techniques to facilitate positive change. Gradually deepening the trance through relaxation techniques or by using progressive suggestions over time can also help the subject reach deeper states of hypnosis.

Hypnosis, like any therapeutic method, is not a one-size-fits-all solution. There are various reasons why hypnosis may not work as effectively in some cases, including resistance, unrealistic expectations, physical discomfort, and mental health conditions. By understanding these limitations and adapting your approach, you can maximize the chances of a successful session. It is important to recognize when hypnosis is not the right tool for a particular situation and, if necessary, refer the subject to the appropriate professional care. Ultimately, patience, communication, and an understanding of each individual's needs are key to successful hypnosis practice.

Recognizing and Addressing Negative Reactions
What to Do if Someone Reacts Badly to Hypnosis
While hypnosis is generally safe and effective for many people, there can be occasions where a subject may have a negative reaction. These reactions, while rare, can vary in severity and may manifest during or after the session. Recognizing these reactions and knowing how to address them is an essential part of being a responsible hypnotist.

1. Signs of Negative Reactions
Recognizing negative reactions early can help you manage the situation effectively and ensure the safety and comfort of your subject.

- *Physical Discomfort*: Some subjects may experience feelings of dizziness, nausea, or a sense of heaviness or lightness during hypnosis. This can be due to the body's physical response to deep relaxation or stress.
- *Anxiety or Panic*: Though rare, some individuals may experience heightened anxiety or panic during a session. This can be triggered by fears of losing control or by anxiety about the hypnosis process itself.
- *Emotional Distress*: In some cases, hypnosis can bring up repressed emotions or memories, which may lead to crying, distress, or discomfort. This is especially true when using techniques like age regression or parts therapy.
- *Confusion or Disorientation*: If a subject is confused or disoriented after the session, they may feel unsettled or unsure about what occurred, even if the session was beneficial.
- *Resistance to Suggestions*: Some individuals may resist or reject suggestions, either consciously or unconsciously, which can cause frustration or hinder progress during the session.

2. Immediate Actions to Take if a Negative Reaction Occurs

If a subject has a negative reaction during or after a session, there are several steps you can take to help them feel more comfortable and safe.

- *Stay Calm and Reassuring:* If the subject shows signs of distress, remain calm and maintain a reassuring tone. Let them know that they are safe and that it's okay to feel uncomfortable. Reassure them that they are in control and can end the session at any time.
  - Example: "It's okay to feel this way. You are in a safe place, and you are completely in control. We can slow things down or stop if you need to."
- *Gently Bring Them Out of Trance:* If the subject is experiencing significant discomfort, it's best to bring them out of the hypnotic state. Use a gentle and gradual technique to return them to full awareness. This will help reduce confusion and bring them back to a relaxed, alert state.
  - Example: "I'm going to count you back to full awareness. With each number, you'll feel more awake and alert. One... slowly coming back... Two... feeling more aware... Three... fully awake, feeling refreshed."
- *Offer Reassurance and Support:* After bringing the subject out of the trance, ask how they are feeling. Allow them to express any emotions or discomfort they might have. If they are confused or disoriented, provide further reassurance, and let them know that their experience was normal, but that you can adjust the process for future sessions.
- *Dealing with Emotional Reactions:* If the subject becomes emotionally distressed or begins to cry, allow them to process their emotions in a safe space. Let them know it's okay to release feelings, and give them time to regain composure. Sometimes, emotional reactions during hypnosis can be a form of catharsis, where repressed emotions surface for healing.
  - Example: "It's okay to cry or feel upset. You're releasing old emotions, and it's a healthy part of the process. Take your time, and we can talk when you're ready."
- *Addressing Anxiety and Panic:* If the subject begins to feel anxious or

panicked during the session, it's important to guide them through it. Use grounding techniques or calming words to help them regain their focus. Gently remind them of their control over the process and offer to stop if necessary.

- ○ Example: "You are completely safe, and you are in control of this process. Let's take some deep breaths together to calm your body and mind."

3. Preventing Negative Reactions in Future Sessions
While some reactions are unavoidable, there are steps you can take to minimize the likelihood of negative reactions in the future:

- *Pre-Session Communication:* Before beginning any hypnosis session, it's important to thoroughly explain the process to your subject. Discuss potential experiences, including any discomfort they might feel, and let them know they are always in control. This helps reduce anxiety and prepares them for what to expect.
    - ○ Example: "During hypnosis, you might experience sensations of relaxation, or even vivid thoughts or emotions. This is all normal, and you will remain in control the entire time."
- *Assess Readiness and Willingness:* Ensure that your subject is truly ready and willing to undergo hypnosis. Ask them about their goals, expectations, and any concerns they may have before starting. If they seem uncertain or apprehensive, take extra time to build rapport and trust.
    - ○ Example: "Are you ready to begin? Do you have any concerns or questions about the process?"
- *Monitor for Resistance:* Throughout the session, watch for signs of resistance, such as tensing of the body, avoidance of eye contact, or verbal hesitations. If you sense resistance, acknowledge it and gently address it. Use calming words and adjust your approach to make the subject more comfortable.
    - ○ Example: "I notice that you seem a bit tense. It's okay to

relax. Let's take a moment to breathe deeply and make sure you feel comfortable."

- *Use Relaxation Techniques:* Before beginning deeper hypnotic work, ensure that your subject is thoroughly relaxed. Use progressive relaxation or other calming techniques to help them ease into the session, making it less likely that they will become overwhelmed.
- *Tailor Sessions to the Individual:* Different people respond to hypnosis in different ways. Some subjects may be more suggestible, while others may require longer inductions or deeper rapport-building. Adjust your approach to the specific needs of the individual.
- *Know When to Refer*: If a subject repeatedly has negative reactions, despite your best efforts, it may be an indication that hypnosis is not the right approach for them at this time. If the person is dealing with complex psychological or emotional issues, it may be appropriate to refer them to a licensed mental health professional.

4. After the Session

Even if the subject had a negative experience during the session, it's important to follow up and provide support.

- *Post-Session Debriefing:* After the session, take time to talk to your subject about what they experienced. Ask them how they felt and whether they encountered any discomfort or distress. Use this feedback to improve future sessions.
  - Example: "Now that we're finished, how are you feeling? Was there anything that was difficult for you during the session?"
- *Provide Encouragement:* If the subject experienced negative emotions or reactions, offer encouragement. Let them know that it's normal for some people to experience emotional release or discomfort, especially in the beginning stages of therapy.
- *Offer Additional Resources*: If necessary, suggest additional resources such as relaxation techniques, meditation, or further reading to help the subject manage their feelings after the session.

5. When to Seek Professional Help

If a subject continues to experience negative reactions during hypnosis or if they show signs of distress that you cannot manage, it may be necessary to seek professional assistance. Consider referring the subject to a licensed therapist or counselor, especially if the individual is dealing with deep-seated emotional trauma or a psychological condition that requires more specialized treatment.

Negative reactions to hypnosis, though rare, are important to recognize and address quickly to ensure the well-being of the subject. By remaining calm, offering reassurance, and adjusting your approach, you can help guide the subject through any discomfort and foster a more positive experience. Open communication before, during, and after the session is crucial for preventing and managing negative reactions, ensuring that hypnosis remains a safe and effective therapeutic tool.

Conclusion and Next Steps: Summarizing Key Takeaways

As you reach the end of this guidebook, it's important to take a moment to reflect on the key concepts and techniques you've learned. Whether you are just beginning your journey into hypnosis or have been practicing for a while, this chapter serves as a reminder of the core elements that will help you succeed as a hypnotist.

Here's a recap of the essential points from this book:

1. *What Hypnosis Is (and Isn't)*
    - *Hypnosis is a focused, relaxed state where the subconscious mind becomes more receptive to suggestion.*
    - *It is not mind control, nor is it something that causes you to lose complete control. Hypnosis is a cooperative process.*
2. *The Mind and Consciousness*
    - *Understanding the distinction between the conscious and subconscious mind is essential to working with hypnosis.*
    - *The subconscious mind plays a pivotal role in habit change, emotional healing, and behavior modification.*
3. *The Hypnotic State*
    - *Hypnosis involves an altered state of consciousness in which the subject is deeply relaxed and highly suggestible.*
    - *Inductions, such as progressive relaxation or eye fixation, help guide someone into this state. Deepening techniques are then used to enhance the trance.*
4. *Building Rapport and Trust*
    - *Establishing a trusting, respectful relationship is crucial to a successful hypnosis session.*

5. *Hypnotic Induction Techniques*
   ○ *You've learned various ways to induce hypnosis, from progressive relaxation to rapid inductions.*
   ○ *Tailoring the technique to each individual's personality and needs is key to effective hypnosis.*

6. *Deepening the Trance*
   ○ *Deepening techniques, such as visualizations or countdowns, help enhance the subject's hypnotic state.*
   ○ *Recognizing signs of deep hypnosis will allow you to gauge when the subject is most receptive to suggestions.*

7. *Hypnotic Suggestions*
   ○ *Suggestions are the heart of hypnosis. You've learned how to craft clear, effective suggestions that are designed to be positive, specific, and helpful.*
   ○ *You also learned to deal with resistance and how to apply indirect or post-hypnotic suggestions to address deeper issues.*

8. *Applications of Hypnosis*
   ○ *Hypnosis can be used in a wide range of areas, from therapeutic applications (e.g., pain management, stress relief) to personal development and performance enhancement.*
   ○ *You've learned that hypnosis can be a powerful tool for overcoming bad habits, enhancing confidence, and promoting relaxation.*

9. *Advanced Techniques*
   ○ *You've explored advanced techniques such as Parts Therapy, Age Regression, and Cognitive Restructuring, which can address deep-rooted psychological issues.*
   ○ *Techniques like confusion and Ericksonian methods provide you with tools for inducing hypnosis in creative, conversational ways.*

10. *Ethical Considerations*
   ○ *Ethics are a critical part of being a responsible hypnotist. Always respect your subject's autonomy, and ensure you have*

informed consent before performing hypnosis.
- ○ *Recognizing the limits of hypnosis and avoiding overstepping professional boundaries are essential for your credibility and the subject's well-being.*

11. *Practical Sessions and Case Studies*
    - ○ *You've seen real-life examples of hypnosis in action. These case studies helped demonstrate how to apply techniques and troubleshoot any issues that arise in a session.*

12. *Self-Improvement for the Hypnotist*
    - ○ *The best hypnotists are those who continually strive to improve their skills.*
    - ○ *Practicing regularly, reflecting on your sessions, and seeking feedback from others will help you become more proficient.*

13. *Troubleshooting and Problem Solving*
    - ○ *You've learned how to deal with difficult subjects, how to manage resistance, and how to troubleshoot issues that may arise during sessions.*

Next Steps: Moving Forward in Your Hypnosis Practice

As you continue your journey into the world of hypnosis, here are some next steps to help you grow and refine your skills:

1. *Practice, Practice, Practice*
    - ○ *The more you practice hypnosis, the more confident and skilled you'll become. Begin practicing with friends, family, or volunteers, ensuring that you're creating a safe, comfortable environment.*

2. *Keep Learning*
    - ○ *Hypnosis is a vast field with continuous advancements. Seek out additional books, courses, and seminars to deepen your knowledge.*
    - ○ *Learn from experienced professionals, and if possible, find a mentor who can guide you on your path.*

3. *Experiment with Different Techniques*
    - ○ *Not every subject responds the same way to hypnosis, so try*

different inductions, deepening techniques, and suggestions until you find what works best for each individual.

- *Experiment with advanced techniques like Parts Therapy or Age Regression in a controlled, ethical manner to expand your skill set.*

4. *Build a Professional Practice*
   - *If you're considering using hypnosis in a professional capacity, start by setting up a practice. Research the ethical and legal requirements in your area, and consider gaining certification through a recognized hypnosis organization.*
   - *Building a successful hypnosis practice requires continuous learning, adaptability, and a genuine desire to help others.*

5. *Self-Hypnosis for Personal Growth*
   - *Hypnosis isn't just for working with others—it's also an effective tool for personal development. Continue practicing self-hypnosis to enhance your own confidence, relaxation, and goal-setting abilities.*
   - *Use self-hypnosis to overcome limiting beliefs, reduce stress, and unlock your potential.*

6. *Monitor Your Progress*
   - *As you apply hypnosis in your daily life and with others, keep track of your progress. Record sessions, reflect on what worked, and adjust your approach as necessary.*
   - *Seek feedback from subjects, and be open to learning from both successes and challenges.*

Final Thoughts

Hypnosis is a powerful tool that can be used for transformation, growth, and healing. As you continue to explore and practice the techniques outlined in this book, remember that mastery comes with patience and dedication. It's not just about the techniques but about understanding people and building a connection based on trust and mutual respect.

By following the steps outlined here, staying curious, and committing to ethical practice, you can make a meaningful impact on the lives of others through hypnosis. The journey doesn't end with this book—it is only the beginning.

Keep practicing, learning, and growing, and you'll be well on your way to becoming a confident, skilled hypnotist.

Good luck on your journey, and may hypnosis help you and those you work with achieve great things!

This concludes the guidebook, but your learning and practice are just beginning. Best of luck!

PART 2: CASE STUDIES

Practical Sessions and Case Studies

Demonstrating a Hypnosis Session: Step-by-Step Walkthroughs of Real-Life Hypnosis Sessions

In this chapter, we will explore the practical application of hypnosis by providing detailed, step-by-step walkthroughs of real-life hypnosis sessions. This will help demystify the process for both beginners and experienced hypnotists, showcasing how to apply the techniques, theories, and skills learned in previous chapters. By examining different types of hypnosis sessions, we will understand how to tailor your approach to the needs of each individual subject. We will walk through a typical session, from pre-session preparation to the post-session debriefing, as well as explore a variety of real-life case studies. These sessions will highlight different approaches, challenges, and techniques used in various settings, such as therapeutic hypnosis, performance enhancement, and relaxation.

1. Pre-Session Preparation: Setting Up for Success

Before starting any hypnosis session, it is essential to set the stage properly to ensure that the subject feels safe, comfortable, and ready to engage in the process. The environment should be calm, quiet, and free of distractions, allowing the subject to relax fully.

Key Steps in Pre-Session Preparation:

- *Create a Comfortable Environment:* Ensure the room is quiet, dimly lit, and free from distractions. Use comfortable chairs or seating for the subject, and make sure the temperature is conducive to relaxation.

- *Establish Trust:* Begin by discussing the goals of the session with the subject. Review their expectations, clarify any questions, and reassure them that they are in control throughout the process.

- *Review Consent and Boundaries:* Before beginning the hypnosis session, reiterate the process of informed consent, emphasizing that they can stop the session at any time if they feel uncomfortable. Discuss any specific preferences or boundaries that should be respected during the session.

2. Induction Phase: Guiding the Subject into a Hypnotic State

The induction phase is the beginning of the hypnosis session, where the hypnotist uses various techniques to guide the subject into a relaxed, focused state of heightened suggestibility. Below is a detailed example of a progressive relaxation induction technique.

Step-by-Step: Progressive Relaxation Induction

1. *Start with Relaxation:*
   - *"Take a deep breath in... and as you breathe out, feel your body start to relax. Let go of any tension in your shoulders, arms, and neck."*
   - *Guide the subject to progressively relax each part of their body, from head to toe.*
   - *"Now, imagine a warm wave of relaxation slowly spreading through your body, starting from your head and moving down through your neck, shoulders, arms, and legs."*
2. *Deepening the Relaxation:*
   - *"With each breath, you go deeper into relaxation, feeling your body become lighter and more relaxed with every exhale."*
   - *Use visualizations, such as imagining descending stairs or floating on a cloud, to deepen the trance state.*
3. *Focus the Mind:*
   - *"Focus all your attention on the sound of my voice. If your mind wanders, simply bring it back to my voice, allowing yourself to relax even deeper."*
   - *Maintain a calm, soothing tone to reinforce relaxation and keep the subject's focus.*

3. Deepening the Trance: Enhancing the Hypnotic State

Once the subject has entered a light trance, the hypnotist will deepen the state to increase receptivity to suggestions. Deepening techniques, such as counting down or using visual imagery, are used to achieve this.

Step-by-Step: Counting Down for Deeper Trance

1. *Counting Method:*
   - *"I'm going to count from 10 to 1. With each number, you'll feel yourself relaxing even more deeply, going deeper and deeper into a state of calm and comfort."*
   - *Slowly count down from 10 to 1, pausing after each number to allow the subject to feel progressively deeper relaxation.*
2. *Use of Imagery:*
   - *"As you continue to relax, imagine yourself descending down a beautiful staircase, each step bringing you closer to a peaceful, calm state. With every step, you feel more relaxed, more at ease."*
   - *Alternatively, use imagery like sinking into a comfortable chair, lying on a warm beach, or floating on a peaceful lake to facilitate deeper relaxation.*

4. Suggestion Phase: Delivering Positive Hypnotic Suggestions

Once the subject is in a deep trance, the hypnotist can begin delivering suggestions. These suggestions are intended to help the subject achieve the goals of the session, whether for therapeutic, performance, or relaxation purposes.

Step-by-Step: Crafting and Delivering Suggestions

1. *Therapeutic Suggestions (e.g., Stress Relief):*
   - *"Now that you are deeply relaxed, your mind is open and receptive to positive change. Imagine yourself in a peaceful place, where you feel completely safe and free from stress. Every time you take a deep breath, feel any remaining tension melt away."*
   - *Reinforce the idea that the subject is in control and that they can bring this sense of relaxation and calm into their everyday*

life.

2. *Behavioral Suggestions (e.g., Habit Change):*
    - *"In your mind, see yourself making healthy choices and feeling empowered to say no to habits that no longer serve you. Each time you make a choice that is in alignment with your goals, you feel proud and more confident."*
    - *Frame the suggestion in positive, future-focused language to encourage lasting change.*
3. *Post-Hypnotic Suggestions:*
    - *"After this session, you will feel more relaxed and at ease every time you encounter a stressful situation. You will carry this sense of calm with you throughout your day."*

5. Awakening Phase: Bringing the Subject Out of Trance

At the end of the session, it is important to gently bring the subject out of trance and help them return to a fully alert state. This is often done by gradually counting up, bringing the subject's awareness back to the present moment.

Step-by-Step: Awakening the Subject

1. *Gradual Counting Up:*
    - *"I'm going to count from 1 to 5, and as I do, you will become more aware of your surroundings, feeling more awake and alert with each number."*
    - *Start at 1, giving the subject time to process each step, and gradually bring them back to full awareness.*
2. *Reassurance:*
    - *"As you open your eyes and come back to full awareness, know that you feel refreshed, relaxed, and alert, carrying the calm energy with you throughout your day."*
    - *Reinforce positive feelings and remind the subject of any post-hypnotic suggestions given during the session.*

6. Post-Session Debriefing and Follow-Up

After the session, it's essential to have a debriefing to ensure the subject feels comfortable, discuss any sensations or feelings that may have arisen during the session, and reinforce the positive effects of the hypnosis.

Step-by-Step: Post-Session Debriefing

1. *Ask About Their Experience:*
   - *"How are you feeling now? What was your experience like during the session?"*
   - *Provide space for the subject to reflect on the session and share any emotions or thoughts.*
2. *Reinforce Positive Changes:*
   - *"You've made great progress today, and you'll continue to feel more relaxed and in control as you carry these positive changes forward."*
   - *If appropriate, schedule follow-up sessions to monitor progress and deepen the work.*
3. *Offer Additional Resources:*
   - *If the subject is working on a specific issue, provide resources, such as relaxation techniques or journaling exercises, to support the process between sessions.*

7. Case Studies: Real-Life Applications of Hypnosis

To illustrate the versatility and effectiveness of hypnosis, we'll explore a few real-life case studies demonstrating different types of hypnosis sessions and their outcomes. These examples will highlight how hypnosis can be tailored to suit the unique needs of each subject, showcasing both therapeutic and performance-related applications.

Case Study 1: Overcoming Smoking Habit

- *Goal*: Help a subject quit smoking using hypnosis to break the behavioral pattern.
- *Approach*: The subject was guided through a progressive relaxation induction, followed by post-hypnotic suggestions to reinforce a new identity as a non-smoker. The suggestions included visualizations of the subject enjoying healthy activities, such as exercising or socializing

without smoking.

- *Outcome*: After several sessions, the subject successfully reduced and ultimately eliminated their smoking habit, reporting fewer cravings and a heightened sense of well-being.

Case Study 2: Enhancing Confidence for Public Speaking

- *Goal*: Increase confidence in a subject's ability to speak publicly without fear.
- *Approach*: A combination of deepening techniques, visualizations, and positive affirmations were used to help the subject reframe their fear of public speaking. The hypnotist guided them to imagine speaking in front of a supportive audience, with feelings of calm and confidence growing as they spoke.
- *Outcome*: The subject reported increased confidence and decreased anxiety before and during public speaking events, leading to better performances and a reduction in stage fright.

Case Study 3: Managing Chronic Pain

- *Goal*: Use hypnosis to help a subject manage chronic pain due to arthritis.
- *Approach*: The subject was guided into a deep trance using a progressive relaxation technique. After deepening, the hypnotist gave suggestions to reduce pain perception, visualizing the pain as a manageable, dissipating sensation.
- *Outcome*: The subject experienced a significant reduction in pain intensity and reported feeling more in control of their pain management.

Through real-life case studies and detailed, step-by-step walkthroughs, this chapter provides readers with a practical understanding of how to conduct a hypnosis session. By following these processes and adapting techniques to the needs of each subject, you can apply hypnosis in various settings to achieve therapeutic, performance, or relaxation goals.

Analyzing Case Studies: Examples of Successful Hypnosis Sessions and What to Learn from Them

In this section, we will examine several real-world case studies of hypnosis sessions, highlighting their objectives, techniques used, challenges faced, and the outcomes achieved. By analyzing these cases, we can better understand how hypnosis can be applied to various situations and what techniques were most effective in each case. We will also discuss what you can learn from these case studies to improve your own practice and enhance your understanding of hypnosis.

Case Study 1: Overcoming Smoking Addiction

Objective:

The goal of this session was to help a subject, a 35-year-old woman, quit smoking after years of dependence.

Techniques Used:

- *Induction*: The session began with a progressive relaxation induction to help the subject achieve a deep state of relaxation. This was followed by the eye fixation method to deepen the trance.
- *Deepening*: The hypnotist used a countdown technique, starting from 10 to 1, to increase the subject's level of relaxation and focus.
- *Suggestions*: Positive, future-oriented suggestions were given, reinforcing the idea that the subject could live without cigarettes. The hypnotist used post-hypnotic suggestions such as: "Whenever you feel the urge to smoke, you will feel a sense of calm and choose to take a deep breath instead."
- *Visualization*: The subject was guided to visualize herself in social situations, feeling confident and free from the need to smoke.

Challenges Faced:

- *Deep-rooted Habit:* The subject had been smoking for 15 years, and the habit was deeply ingrained in her daily routine. Overcoming such a long-standing behavior required patience and persistence.

- *Resistance*: At first, the subject resisted the idea that she could stop smoking easily, expressing doubt about her ability to change.

Outcome:

- After the first session, the subject experienced a significant reduction in cravings. She reported feeling empowered and in control of her actions. By the third session, she had quit smoking entirely, and continued to report no desire to return to the habit. Follow-up sessions were scheduled to reinforce the changes.

Lessons Learned:

- *Reinforcement is Key:* With behaviors like smoking, it is essential to provide consistent reinforcement through positive suggestions and visualization. This helps to replace the old behavior with a healthier alternative.
- *Patience and Persistence*: Long-standing habits require time and persistence to overcome. Even if initial results are not immediate, gradual change can still lead to success.

Case Study 2: Performance Enhancement for Public Speaking

Objective:

The subject, a 28-year-old man, sought help to overcome his fear of public speaking and boost his confidence before an important presentation at work.

Techniques Used:

- *Induction*: The session began with a progressive relaxation technique, followed by deepening through guided imagery. The subject was asked to imagine descending a staircase, each step taking him deeper into relaxation.
- *Suggestions*: The hypnotist gave positive affirmations such as: "You are confident, calm, and clear when speaking in front of others."

Additionally, future-paced *suggestions* were introduced, imagining the subject delivering his presentation effortlessly and with confidence.

- *Visualization*: The subject was guided to vividly imagine himself in front of his audience, smiling, speaking clearly, and feeling relaxed as he engaged with the crowd.
- *Anchoring*: The hypnotist used an anchoring technique, asking the subject to associate a gesture (e.g., touching his thumb and forefinger together) with feelings of calm and confidence during his presentation.

Challenges Faced:

- *Deep-rooted Anxiety:* The subject had a long history of fear and anxiety around public speaking, which resulted in a significant amount of resistance during the initial stages of the session.
- *Negative Self-Talk*: The subject had a tendency to ruminate on past failures and negative experiences, which created mental blocks that made it hard to visualize success.

Outcome:

- After the first session, the subject reported feeling much calmer and more confident in his daily interactions. By the time of the presentation, he was able to speak confidently in front of his audience, receiving positive feedback from colleagues.
- Follow-up sessions reinforced the new, positive mindset and helped eliminate any lingering anxiety before future public speaking engagements.

Lessons Learned:

- *Visualization and Positive Affirmations:* Visualization techniques combined with positive affirmations are powerful tools for boosting confidence. The more vivid and sensory-rich the visualizations, the more effective they are at creating lasting changes.

- *Rewriting the Narrative:* Addressing negative self-talk and past failures is essential for overcoming performance anxiety. Helping the subject reframe their narrative and envision future success can break the cycle of fear.

Case Study 3: Managing Chronic Pain

Objective:

A 50-year-old man, who had been suffering from chronic back pain due to an old injury, sought relief through hypnosis. The pain had become debilitating and was not responsive to medical treatment.

Techniques Used:

- *Induction*: The session began with a deep progressive relaxation technique, with an emphasis on relaxing the back muscles.
- *Deepening*: The hypnotist deepened the trance using breathing techniques and visualizations, encouraging the subject to imagine himself in a peaceful place, like a beach or garden, where he felt completely at ease.
- *Pain Control Suggestions:* The hypnotist gave direct suggestions to alter the pain perception: "With every breath, the pain in your back becomes less and less, as if it is slowly melting away." The subject was encouraged to visualize the pain as a color or object that could be transformed or removed.
- *Anchor Creation:* The subject was taught to use an anchoring technique to activate pain relief. By touching his thumb and forefinger together, he could trigger the relaxation and pain relief response.

Challenges Faced:

- *Skepticism*: The subject was initially skeptical of hypnosis and doubted its effectiveness in alleviating his physical pain. He also had a history of chronic pain and was accustomed to living with discomfort.

- *Pain Intensity*: The pain was quite intense, and although the initial session provided some relief, it took several sessions to achieve a significant reduction.

Outcome:

- After the third session, the subject reported a noticeable reduction in pain, experiencing periods of complete relief. He was able to engage in activities that had previously been too painful, such as walking and gardening. The subject continued to practice self-hypnosis techniques on his own between sessions.

Lessons Learned:

- *Gradual Relief:* In cases of chronic pain, it is important to manage expectations. While hypnosis can be highly effective, pain reduction may require multiple sessions and a gradual approach.
- *Self-Hypnosis for Long-Term Results:* Teaching the subject self-hypnosis techniques empowers them to manage pain on their own, allowing for greater long-term relief and autonomy.
- *Visualization and Reframing:* In pain management, visualization and reframing are essential tools for changing the way the brain processes discomfort.

Case Study 4: Overcoming Insomnia

Objective:

A 42-year-old woman who had been struggling with insomnia for over a year sought help to regain restful sleep.

Techniques Used:

- *Induction*: The session began with a progressive muscle relaxation technique, followed by gentle suggestions to induce sleepiness.
- *Deepening*: Deepening was achieved using a countdown technique, with the subject imagining herself sinking deeper into a comfortable, restful state with each count.

- *Suggestions*: The hypnotist used positive sleep suggestions, such as: "Every night, you will find it easy to fall asleep, and you will sleep deeply and restfully through the night."
- *Visualization*: The subject was guided to imagine a calm, serene scene—such as lying in a hammock on a quiet beach—helping her body and mind associate these peaceful images with the act of falling asleep.

Challenges Faced:

- *Conditioned Insomnia:* The subject had developed conditioned insomnia, where the anticipation of sleeplessness triggered anxiety and further disrupted sleep patterns.
- *Stress and Anxiety*: Underlying anxiety from work and personal life exacerbated the insomnia, making it harder for her to unwind before bedtime.

Outcome:

- After three sessions, the subject experienced a marked improvement in sleep quality, with fewer interruptions during the night and quicker onset of sleep. By the fifth session, the subject reported consistently sleeping through the night without difficulty.
- The subject continued to use relaxation techniques before bed to reinforce the positive sleep patterns.

Lessons Learned:

- *Relaxation is Crucial:* For insomnia, relaxation is a key component in promoting sleep. Techniques like progressive relaxation, deep breathing, and visualization are essential to calm both the body and mind.
- *Addressing Underlying Stress:* Insomnia often has underlying psychological causes, such as stress and anxiety. These need to be addressed during hypnosis sessions to ensure long-term improvement.

- *Reinforcement Through Regular Sessions*: Insomnia may require a few sessions to break the cycle of sleeplessness, especially when it's rooted in anxiety or stress. Regular reinforcement is key.

Key Takeaways

By analyzing these case studies, we can see the variety of ways hypnosis can be used effectively for different goals—whether overcoming addiction, enhancing performance, managing chronic pain, or improving sleep. Key lessons from these cases include:

- The importance of tailoring techniques to the subject's needs and goals.
- The power of visualization in reinforcing positive change.
- The need for patience and persistence, especially with long-standing issues like addiction or chronic pain.

These case studies provide a practical foundation for anyone interested in learning how to apply hypnosis effectively and ethically.

PART 3: SAMPLE SCRIPTS

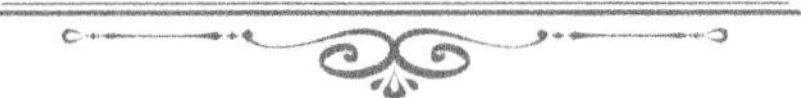

Stress Relief and Relaxation Hypnosis Script

Induction:

"Take a comfortable seat or lie down, and begin to focus on your breathing. Allow yourself to take a deep, slow breath in... and then gently exhale. With each breath you take, you begin to feel more relaxed, more at ease.

Let's take another deep breath in... and slowly breathe out, releasing any tension in your body. As you continue breathing in a slow and steady rhythm, I want you to notice how each breath you take brings you a little bit more relaxation, and with each exhale, you let go of any stress, tension, or worries.

Now, with every breath, feel your body becoming heavier and heavier... as if you are sinking deeper into a comfortable surface, supported and safe.

I'm going to count from 10 to 1. With each number, you will feel yourself becoming more relaxed, and more deeply at ease. Ten... feeling calm and comfortable. Nine... going deeper... Eight... with every breath, you feel yourself relax even more... Seven... every muscle in your body letting go of tension... Six... feeling calmness spreading from your head down to your toes... Five... deepening your relaxation... Four... becoming more and more at ease... Three... feeling completely comfortable... Two... more relaxed now than you have ever felt... And one... deeply relaxed."

Deepening the Relaxation:

"Now, imagine a warm, soothing wave of relaxation gently flowing down from the top of your head. This wave moves slowly, bringing calm and relaxation to every part of your body. As it moves down, it releases any remaining tension you may have, bringing complete relaxation to each area it passes.

The wave moves from your scalp, down to your forehead, softening the muscles in your face. Feel your eyes soften and relax. It flows down to your neck and shoulders, melting away any tension, allowing your body to relax even more deeply.

Feel this warm, soothing wave move down your arms, all the way to your fingertips. Let go of any remaining tension. Now, the wave continues down your chest, down your back, all the way to your stomach, bringing a calmness that makes you feel lighter, more at ease.

The wave continues its journey down to your legs, relaxing your thighs, your knees, and your calves. Finally, the wave moves to your feet, all the way down to your toes. And with that, your entire body is now completely relaxed, calm, and at peace."

Stress Relief Suggestion:

"Now that you're deeply relaxed, I want you to imagine a peaceful place—somewhere where you feel completely calm, safe, and at ease. This might be a beach, a quiet forest, a garden, or any other place where you feel completely relaxed.

In this peaceful place, there is a gentle breeze, or soft sounds that help you relax even more. You can feel the warmth of the sun or hear the rustling of leaves. Everything around you feels soothing, and you feel a sense of deep tranquility.

As you take in the peaceful atmosphere of this place, I want you to notice that in your hand, you're holding a small, imaginary container—perhaps a box or a jar. You are holding all of the stress and tension that you've been carrying. This container has the ability to hold all of your worries, your frustrations, and the pressure you've been feeling.

As you look at this container, you notice that it is now beginning to absorb all of the stress and tension you've been holding. The container takes in all of those negative feelings, and with each breath you take, more and more of that stress is drawn into the container, leaving your body and mind feeling lighter and more at ease.

Take a deep breath in... and as you exhale, feel even more stress leaving your body, flowing into the container. You may notice your body becoming more relaxed with every breath. Let the container hold onto all of that stress for you, as you continue to breathe deeply and comfortably.

And now, when you feel ready, you can set that container down, knowing it is holding all the stress and tension, and you can walk away from it—free from its weight. You leave all the pressure and negativity behind, and you feel lighter, more relaxed, and more at peace."

Affirmations for Stress Relief:

"From this moment forward, whenever you begin to feel stress or tension, you will automatically remember this peaceful place, and you will find yourself feeling calm and at ease. Your body knows how to relax, and every time you take a deep breath, you will find yourself returning to this feeling of tranquility and peace. You are in control, and you can let go of stress easily whenever you choose.

You have the power to remain calm, focused, and at peace, no matter what challenges arise in your life. Stress no longer has control over you. You are calm, confident, and capable of handling any situation with ease."

Awakening:

"Now, it's time to return to full awareness, bringing with you this sense of peace and relaxation. In a moment, I will count from 1 to 5. With each number, you will become more alert, more aware of your surroundings, and feeling refreshed, calm, and rejuvenated. One... slowly bringing your awareness back... Two... feeling more alert, and more awake... Three... noticing the energy returning to your body... Four... you are calm, relaxed, and refreshed... Five... fully awake now, feeling alert, clear, and at peace."

This script provides a comprehensive session focused on stress relief and relaxation. You can adjust the imagery and suggestions based on the specific needs of the subject or the type of relaxation you're aiming to achieve. This script could also be used for self-hypnosis practice.

Next is a full hypnosis script for *Overcoming Bad Habits*, specifically for *overeating*. This script will focus on helping the subject develop a healthier relationship with food, increase control over eating habits, and promote mindful eating.

Overcoming Overeating Hypnosis Script

Induction:

"Make yourself comfortable and take a deep breath in... hold it for a moment... and then exhale slowly, letting go of any tension. With each breath you take, you feel your body becoming more relaxed, more at ease.

Take another deep breath in... and breathe out slowly, releasing any stress, any worries, and any tension in your body. With each breath, you feel more and more relaxed. Your mind is quieting down, your body is softening, and you are beginning to feel calm and peaceful.

As you continue breathing deeply and steadily, I want you to allow yourself to let go of anything that isn't serving you right now. With every breath, you release tension and open yourself up to positive change.

I will now count from 10 to 1. With each number, you will become more deeply relaxed, sinking further into a state of calm and peace. Ten... feeling relaxed and at ease. Nine... deeper still. Eight... your body becoming heavier, more comfortable. Seven... every breath you take relaxes you even more. Six... your mind is calm and peaceful. Five... sinking deeper with every breath. Four... feeling more and more relaxed. Three... you're going deeper into relaxation now. Two... every muscle is loose, comfortable, and at ease. One... you're deeply relaxed now."

Deepening the Relaxation:

"Now that you're feeling so calm and relaxed, I want you to imagine a peaceful place. This could be a garden, a quiet beach, or any place where you feel completely at ease. Imagine yourself there now, feeling the calm energy of this space surrounding you.

As you take in the beauty and peace of this place, you notice that it's filled with soothing sounds, gentle breezes, or comforting scents. Everything here is calm, safe, and peaceful.

As you breathe in this peaceful atmosphere, you can feel any remaining tension or worry melting away. You are calm, comfortable, and completely relaxed. And in this deeply relaxed state, you're ready to make positive, lasting changes."

Addressing Overeating and Creating New Habits:

"Now, while you're in this deeply relaxed state, I want you to think about your relationship with food. Notice any patterns, any moments when you have eaten more than you needed. You may not be consciously aware of all of them, but you can allow yourself to recognize them now. And as you notice these patterns, I want you to understand that it's okay—this is simply an old habit, one that no longer serves you.

As you stand in your peaceful place, I want you to picture a glowing light in front of you. This light represents your healthy, balanced relationship with food. This light is filled with positive energy, self-control, and mindful eating. It's warm and inviting, and it feels good to be near it.

As you move closer to this light, feel its energy fill you with a sense of control and understanding. You understand that food is not just for comfort; it is fuel for your body. And as you continue to focus on this light, you begin to notice how you feel about food—your desire for healthy, nourishing meals is stronger than any urge to overeat.

From now on, whenever you feel the urge to overeat, you will notice a subtle shift inside of you. You will naturally feel a desire to eat in moderation, to listen to your body's cues, and to stop when you are satisfied—not when you are full. You will find yourself choosing food that nourishes your body and supports your well-being.

Your body knows how to be healthy, and you can trust it. You can trust yourself to make healthy, balanced choices at every meal.

Whenever you're faced with a situation where overeating might be tempting, you will find yourself thinking twice before reaching for food that you don't need. You will listen to your body's signals—its natural cues for hunger, fullness, and satisfaction. You will find it easy to make decisions that support your health and well-being."

Affirmations for Overcoming Overeating:

"From this moment forward, you will find that your desire for healthy, nourishing food will increase, and the urges to overeat will fade away. You will feel in control of your choices. Every time you make a decision about food, it will be a conscious choice, and it will feel good.

You are no longer driven by emotional eating. You will notice that when you're feeling stressed or emotional, you will handle those feelings in a healthier way—not with food, but with other tools that bring you peace, like breathing, mindfulness, or relaxation.

You feel a sense of pride and accomplishment each time you make a choice that supports your health. Every meal, every snack, is a step toward a healthier you."

Awakening:

"Now, I'm going to count from 1 to 5. With each number, you will gradually return to full awareness, bringing with you the positive changes and new habits that you have created. You will return feeling calm, focused, and in control of your eating habits. One... becoming aware of the room around you. Two... gently bringing your awareness back. Three... feeling the energy returning to your body. Four... noticing how refreshed, relaxed, and empowered you feel. And five... fully awake now, feeling alert, calm, and ready to continue making healthy, balanced choices with food."

This script is designed to address overeating by focusing on the emotional and habitual aspects of the behavior. It aims to replace old habits with new, positive ones, helping the subject create a healthier relationship with food. You can personalize this script by adding specific images or experiences that resonate with the individual, and adjust the tone or content based on their needs.

Next is a full hypnosis script designed to *boost confidence and self-esteem.* The goal is to help the subject overcome self-doubt, develop positive self-perceptions, and feel empowered in various areas of their life.

Confidence and Self-Esteem Boost Hypnosis Script

Induction:

"Make yourself comfortable now... allow your body to relax... Take a deep breath in, hold it for a moment, and exhale slowly. With each breath, allow yourself to let go of any tension in your body, any stress or discomfort... just let it go.

Take another deep breath in... breathe in peace, calm, and relaxation... and as you breathe out, imagine releasing any negative thoughts or feelings that may be lingering. Feel the weight of the world lift from your shoulders, and know that you are safe, comfortable, and at ease.

Now, I will count down from ten to one. With each number, you will sink deeper into relaxation, letting go more and more with each breath you take. Ten... feeling calm... nine... becoming more and more relaxed... eight... sinking deeper... seven... feeling heavy and comfortable... six... every breath you take relaxes you even more... five... feeling safe, relaxed, and peaceful... four... your body is completely at ease... three... your mind is quiet and clear... two... you're sinking deeply into relaxation... and one... you are now deeply relaxed, calm, and at peace."

Deepening the Relaxation:

"Now that you're deeply relaxed, imagine yourself standing in front of a beautiful mirror. This mirror is different from any other mirror—it reflects the very best version of you, the confident, empowered, capable version of yourself. As you look into this mirror, you see yourself standing tall and proud, radiating self-confidence and strength. You notice how comfortable and calm you are, how you carry yourself with ease. Your posture is strong, your eyes are bright, and you are at peace with yourself.

With every breath you take, you can feel that version of yourself becoming more and more real. You are beginning to realize that the confident, empowered person in the mirror is not just a reflection—it is the true version of who you are inside. You have always had the potential for this confidence, and now you are unlocking it."

Building Confidence and Self-Esteem:

"Now, I want you to focus on a time in your life when you felt confident and strong. Maybe it was a moment when you achieved something great or felt really good about yourself. As you think about this time, notice how good it felt to be confident. Feel that confidence, that sense of accomplishment, and let it fill your entire body.

Let this feeling grow, expanding from your chest, through your arms, your legs, and all the way to your fingertips and toes. Every part of you is now filled with the confidence and strength that you experienced in that moment. You know that feeling of pride and success. You remember how capable and powerful you were at that time, and you realize that this same confidence and strength are inside you right now.

Whenever you need to access this confidence, you will simply think of that moment and allow those feelings to flow through you. The more you practice this, the stronger and more natural it will become.

You are capable of handling any situation with confidence. Whether it's speaking in front of others, meeting new people, or handling challenges in your life, you now have the inner strength and belief in yourself to handle it all. You know that no matter what happens, you are enough. You are worthy. You are strong."

Positive Affirmations:

"I am confident in myself and my abilities.

I am proud of who I am and all that I have accomplished.

I trust in my own judgment and intuition.

I am deserving of success and happiness.

Every day, I become more confident and empowered.

I believe in myself and my limitless potential."

"Repeat these affirmations in your mind, and as you say them, feel the truth of them deep within your being. Let them resonate throughout your entire body and mind. You are worthy of confidence, and every time you repeat these affirmations, you will feel your self-esteem growing stronger and stronger."

Releasing Limiting Beliefs:

"Now, I want you to think about any limiting beliefs or doubts you may have had about yourself. These could be thoughts like 'I'm not good enough,' or 'I can't do this.' Acknowledge these beliefs for what they are—just old, untrue stories you've told yourself.

As you stand in front of that mirror, picture these limiting beliefs as dark clouds around you. You may notice them, but you can now see them clearly for what they are—just thoughts that no longer serve you.

Now, with each breath, you can feel those clouds disappearing, dissolving into nothingness. The confidence and strength within you are pushing them away, and you are left standing tall and proud, fully aware of your own worth and potential.

You release all of the doubts and fears that have held you back, and you replace them with the unwavering belief that you can do anything you set your mind to."

Awakening:

"Now, I'm going to count from one to five. With each number, you will begin to return to full awareness, bringing with you the new confidence, self-belief, and positive energy that you have gained today. One... feeling more awake, more alert... Two... slowly returning to the present moment... Three... bringing back all the positive energy and confidence you've created... Four... feeling refreshed, empowered, and confident... and Five... fully awake now, eyes open, feeling confident, strong, and ready to take on the world."

This script is designed to enhance confidence and self-esteem by focusing on the subject's past positive experiences, reinforcing empowering beliefs, and removing any limiting thoughts or beliefs that may be holding them back. You can personalize the script further based on the individual's specific needs and goals.

Next is a *full pain management hypnosis script,* designed to help a subject reduce or manage pain by using relaxation, visualization, and suggestion techniques.

Pain Management Hypnosis Script

Induction:

"Make yourself comfortable now... Take a moment to adjust your position, ensuring that you're sitting or lying down in a relaxed way. Gently close your eyes, and take a deep, slow breath in... hold it for a moment... and exhale slowly. Let all tension begin to melt away as you breathe out. With each breath you take, allow your body to relax deeper and deeper.

Take another deep breath in... breathe in calm, peace, and relaxation... and as you breathe out, imagine letting go of any discomfort, stress, or tightness in your body. Feel your muscles releasing all their tension, and with each breath, you are becoming more and more relaxed.

Now, I'm going to count down from ten to one. With each number, you will relax even deeper. Ten... feeling calm... Nine... letting go of all tension... Eight... sinking into a peaceful, deep relaxation... Seven... your body and mind are at ease... Six... feeling more and more relaxed with every breath... Five... allowing yourself to relax even further... Four... peaceful and calm... Three... deepening the relaxation... Two... sinking into a state of total comfort... and One... now completely relaxed, calm, and at peace."

Deepening the Relaxation:

"As you continue to relax, imagine a warm, soothing sensation spreading across your body, from the top of your head down to the tips of your toes. This warmth brings comfort, relaxation, and healing. As the warmth flows, it moves through your forehead... your face... your neck... down through your shoulders, arms, and hands... relaxing and soothing every muscle it touches.

Feel this warm sensation moving down through your chest, your back, your abdomen... allowing every part of your body to relax completely. The warmth flows down through your legs, knees, and all the way to your feet... soothing every muscle, every nerve, every cell. Your entire body is now filled with a gentle, soothing warmth, and you feel peaceful, relaxed, and calm."

Pain Visualization:

"Now, I want you to bring your attention to the area of discomfort in your body. Don't worry, you are in control, and you are completely safe. As you focus on that area, just notice the sensation there… it might feel tight, achy, or uncomfortable. Whatever it feels like, acknowledge it for what it is—just a signal from your body.

Now, I want you to imagine that pain as a color or shape. It might be a bright color, a sharp shape, or something that stands out to you. Picture it clearly in your mind.

Now, imagine that you have a special tool that can change the color, shape, or size of the pain. With every breath you take, imagine that this tool is helping you transform the pain. As you breathe in, you can feel the pain start to dissolve, becoming lighter, softer, and less intense. As you breathe out, imagine it fading away, becoming smaller, weaker, and more distant.

With each breath, you have more and more control over this sensation, and it begins to change to a more neutral or pleasant feeling. You may even begin to notice that the area of discomfort is becoming warmer, softer, or more relaxed. The intensity of the pain is reducing with each breath."

Creating Comfort and Healing:

"Now, imagine a healing light or energy surrounding the area of discomfort. This light is warm, soothing, and healing. It can be any color you prefer—perhaps a soft golden light or a calming blue. As this healing light surrounds the area, it brings comfort, healing, and relaxation.

Feel the energy flowing through your body, bringing relief and comfort to every cell. With each breath, this healing light becomes stronger, soothing any remaining discomfort. The light is now working to heal and restore, bringing balance and relaxation to the area.

Feel this healing energy filling every part of your body, moving through the muscles, nerves, and tissues, soothing and calming the pain completely. As the light continues to work, you feel more and more at ease, and the pain is becoming less and less significant."

Positive Affirmations for Pain Relief:

"Now, repeat the following statements in your mind, allowing the words to sink in deeply:

- My body is capable of healing itself.
- I am in control of my pain, and I can reduce it whenever I choose.
- Each breath I take helps my body heal and relax.
- I am becoming more comfortable, more at ease with each moment.
- I trust my body's ability to heal and restore balance.
- The discomfort is fading, and I am now filled with comfort and ease."

"With every affirmation, notice how much more relaxed and comfortable you become. Feel the pain continue to dissipate with each passing moment, and allow yourself to believe in your body's ability to heal."

Future Pain Management:

"Whenever you need to manage pain or discomfort in the future, you can use this same process. You will remember the warmth, the soothing light, and your ability to change the sensation of discomfort. You have the power to control pain and bring comfort to your body anytime you need it.

From this moment on, whenever you feel discomfort, you can use your mind and body to help reduce or eliminate it. You can breathe deeply, visualize the healing light, and use your tool to transform any discomfort into relaxation. This ability is now a part of you, and it will become easier and more effective each time you practice."

Awakening:

"In a moment, I'm going to count from one to five. With each number, you will begin to return to full awareness, bringing back with you a sense of calm, relaxation, and relief. One... beginning to become more alert... Two... feeling peaceful and relaxed... Three... bringing back the comfort and healing you've experienced... Four... more awake now, refreshed, and at ease... and Five... fully awake now, eyes open, feeling relaxed, empowered, and pain-free."

This script uses a combination of relaxation techniques, visualization, and positive affirmations to help reduce pain. The focus is on empowering the subject with the ability to manage and control their own discomfort. It's important that the subject believes in their ability to influence their pain levels with their mind, and this script helps to instill that confidence. You can modify the script depending on the subject's individual needs or preferences.

Next is a full *overcoming fear hypnosis script,* designed to help a subject confront and reduce fear or anxiety, empowering them to face and overcome their fears in a safe and controlled way.

Overcoming Fear Hypnosis Script

Induction:

"Take a moment now to get comfortable... finding a position where your body can relax fully. Gently close your eyes... and take a deep breath in... filling your lungs with fresh, clean air... hold it for a moment... and then exhale slowly, letting go of any tension or stress.

With each breath you take, feel your body becoming more and more relaxed... breathe in calm, peaceful energy... and breathe out any tension, stress, or discomfort. Feel your muscles begin to loosen, your mind begin to calm.

Now, as you continue to breathe slowly and deeply, I'm going to count down from ten to one. With each number, you will drift deeper and deeper into relaxation... Ten... feeling calm... Nine... more and more at ease... Eight... every muscle relaxing... Seven... your mind becoming calm and peaceful... Six... letting go of the day... Five... sinking deeper... Four... more and more relaxed... Three... deeper still... Two... peaceful, calm, and at ease... and One... deeply relaxed, completely at peace."

Deepening the Relaxation:

"Now, as you continue to relax, imagine a warm, soothing light surrounding your entire body. It's a gentle light, glowing softly, bringing warmth, comfort, and relaxation. Picture this light moving from the top of your head, down to your neck, shoulders, and arms, gently easing away any tension.

Feel this warm light spreading down your back, chest, abdomen, and legs, all the way down to the tips of your toes. With each breath, feel this soothing light relaxing your body even more. Your entire body is now filled with comfort, peace, and tranquility. You are safe, relaxed, and completely at ease."

Addressing the Fear:

"Now, I want you to bring your attention to the fear or anxiety that you've been feeling. You don't need to worry, because in this relaxed state, you are completely safe, and you are in control. Just notice the fear, without judgment, and see it for what it is.

It might be a feeling in your body, a picture, or a sensation. Just notice what it feels like. Allow yourself to become aware of this fear, but remember, you are in control. You are safe, and you have the power to change how you feel about this fear.

Now, imagine this fear as a shape, a color, or an image. What does it look like? What size is it? What color is it? See it clearly in your mind's eye. You may notice that it has a certain texture, or even a sound. Acknowledge it for what it is, without fear, and remember that you have the ability to change it."

Transforming the Fear:

"Now that you've identified the fear, I want you to imagine a powerful, positive force—something that brings you comfort and calm—entering your body. It could be a warm light, a peaceful sound, or even a feeling of strength and courage. As this positive force enters your body, feel it filling you up, moving through your chest, down to your stomach, and into every cell of your body.

This force is powerful, soothing, and completely in control. With every breath you take, this calming, healing energy grows stronger, and it begins to surround the fear. As it does, the fear begins to shrink, becoming smaller and smaller. You can feel the fear softening, losing its grip on you.

The more you breathe in calm and peace, the more the fear fades away. It becomes lighter, softer, and easier to handle. Now, visualize the fear becoming so small and insignificant that it no longer holds any power over you. It's so small now, it's almost invisible.

The calm and soothing energy you've created is now replacing the fear, filling the space where the fear once was. You can feel this transformation happening right now. The fear is fading, replaced by confidence, courage, and peace."

Affirmations of Strength:

"As this fear dissolves, I want you to repeat these words in your mind:

- I am safe, calm, and in control.
- Fear no longer holds power over me.
- I have the strength to face any situation with calmness and confidence.
- I am capable of overcoming anything that challenges me.

- Every day, I become more and more confident in my ability to face my fears.
- I trust myself to handle whatever comes my way with peace and strength."

"Let these words sink deeply into your mind. You are strong, confident, and in control. The fear that once bothered you is now gone, replaced by calmness and self-assurance."

Visualization of Future Success:

"Now, I want you to imagine a situation in the future that would normally trigger this fear. Picture yourself in that situation, but notice how different it feels now. You're calm, relaxed, and confident. The fear is no longer present, and instead, you feel empowered, strong, and at ease.

See yourself handling the situation with complete confidence, taking each step with grace and calm. You are able to face the situation without fear, and you feel proud of your ability to remain calm and confident.

Every time you face a situation like this, you will become more and more confident, more and more at ease. You now have the tools to handle your fear whenever it arises, and each time, it will be easier to remain calm and strong."

Awakening:

"In a moment, I'm going to count from one to five. With each number, you will gradually return to full awareness, bringing with you the calm, confidence, and strength you have developed. You will return to full awareness, feeling empowered, at ease, and completely in control.

One... slowly becoming more aware... Two... feeling refreshed, relaxed, and confident... Three... bringing back all the calm, peace, and strength you've created... Four... feeling more alert, awake, and at ease... and Five... fully awake now, eyes open, feeling calm, confident, and completely in control of your fears."

This script uses a combination of relaxation techniques, positive visualization, and affirmations to help the subject address and overcome their fear. The key is to help them realize they are in control of their emotions and that fear can be managed and transformed. This type of script can be adapted for specific fears, but the process of addressing the fear and replacing it with strength and calm is the same.

Next is full *hypnosis script for overcoming insomnia*, aimed at helping a person relax deeply, calm their mind, and develop healthy sleep patterns. This script can be adapted for different individuals and their specific sleep issues.

Overcoming Insomnia Hypnosis Script

Induction:

"Begin by finding a comfortable position, sitting or lying down, allowing your body to settle into a relaxed state. Close your eyes gently and take a deep breath in... hold it for a moment... and now, slowly exhale, letting go of any tension or stress. With each breath, feel more relaxed, more at ease.

Take another deep breath in... and as you exhale, let go of any thoughts or distractions from the day. Feel your body becoming heavier with each breath, more relaxed, more at peace.

Now, as you continue to breathe slowly and deeply, I'm going to count down from ten to one. With each number, you will feel yourself going deeper and deeper into relaxation. Ten... feeling calm... Nine... letting go of any tension... Eight... more and more relaxed... Seven... your body becoming heavier, more relaxed... Six... sinking deeper... Five... calm, peaceful, and at ease... Four... relaxing more and more... Three... deeper still... Two... feeling your body relax completely... and One... deeply relaxed, at peace, and ready for restful sleep."

Deepening the Relaxation:

"Now, as you relax even more deeply, I want you to imagine a warm, comforting light surrounding your entire body. This light is soft and soothing, filling every part of you with warmth and comfort.

Visualize this light moving down from the top of your head, down your neck and shoulders, all the way down your arms, and all the way to your fingertips. As the light travels, feel every muscle, every fiber of your being become more relaxed, more peaceful.

Feel the light moving down your chest, your abdomen, and your legs, all the way to your toes, bringing calm and relaxation to every part of your body. With each breath, the light deepens your relaxation, and you feel more at ease.

Now, imagine this light becoming brighter and warmer, surrounding you completely. You are now in a state of complete relaxation and peace, and your body is ready for deep, restorative sleep."

Addressing Insomnia:

"Now, as you continue to relax, I want you to focus on your mind. Notice any thoughts or worries that may be present, but know that in this relaxed state, you can let them go. These thoughts don't have to control you. You have the ability to quiet your mind and allow your body to rest deeply.

Imagine your mind is like a calm, peaceful lake. The surface of the water is perfectly still, and the water is clear and calm. If any thoughts come into your mind, imagine them as little ripples on the surface of the water. And just as quickly as the ripples appear, they disappear, leaving the water calm and still once more.

With every breath you take, your thoughts become quieter and quieter. You are able to let go of any worries, stress, or distractions. Your mind is calm, and it is ready for peaceful sleep."

Reframing the Relationship with Sleep:

"Now, I want you to imagine that every night, when it's time for sleep, your mind and body automatically know what to do. You know that sleep is natural for you. You feel safe, relaxed, and comfortable every time you go to bed.

Your mind knows that sleep is a time for deep rest and rejuvenation, and your body knows how to easily and naturally fall asleep. Every time you close your eyes, you will feel your body become heavier, more relaxed, and ready for restful, deep sleep.

In the past, perhaps sleep felt elusive or difficult. But now, you are creating new habits, new ways of thinking about sleep, and you know that with each night, it becomes easier and easier to fall asleep, to stay asleep, and to wake up feeling refreshed and energized.

You can now imagine yourself going to bed, feeling relaxed and comfortable. As your head touches the pillow, you feel your body sink into the mattress, your muscles relax deeply, and your mind calm. You can feel the peaceful, natural rhythm of your breathing slowing down, and your body preparing to drift off to sleep.

And as you drift deeper and deeper, the sleep comes easily. You can feel it in your body, in your mind. You are at peace, and sleep is restful and effortless."

Affirmations for Restful Sleep:
"Now, I want you to repeat these words to yourself, either silently or out loud:

- I am at peace with sleep.
- Sleep comes easily and naturally to me.
- Every night, I sleep deeply and wake up feeling refreshed.
- I release all stress and tension before I sleep.
- I have a positive relationship with sleep, and it is always restful.
- I trust my body to guide me into deep, rejuvenating sleep every night."

"Let these words settle into your mind, like gentle waves washing over you. Each time you say them, you will feel more and more relaxed, more and more confident that sleep is easy, natural, and peaceful."

Visualization of Restful Sleep:
"Now, imagine yourself in the near future, going to bed at night, feeling calm and relaxed. Your mind is quiet, and your body is ready for sleep. Picture yourself falling asleep effortlessly, your breathing slow and steady, your body sinking deeper into the mattress, and your mind drifting off into peaceful, deep sleep.

Visualize yourself sleeping soundly, undisturbed, through the entire night. You sleep deeply, with no interruptions, and you wake up in the morning feeling completely refreshed and energized, ready to begin your day with clarity and vitality.

See yourself enjoying this restful sleep every night. The more you practice this, the easier and more natural it becomes."

Awakening:
"In a moment, I'm going to count from one to five. With each number, you will begin to bring yourself back to full awareness, feeling relaxed, refreshed, and ready for deep, restful sleep. When you reach five, you will feel confident that sleep is easy for you and that every night, you will enjoy a peaceful, undisturbed rest.

One... becoming more aware... Two... feeling calm and at peace... Three... bringing back the relaxation and the knowledge that sleep comes easily to you... Four... feeling more awake, energized, and confident in your ability to sleep deeply... and Five... fully awake now, feeling rested and at ease, ready for a peaceful night's sleep."

This script helps the subject to reframe their relationship with sleep, reduce anxiety around it, and visualize the process of falling and staying asleep with ease. It emphasizes relaxation, releasing tension, and programming the mind to embrace sleep as natural and effortless.

Next is a full *hypnosis script for healing the inner child*, which helps the person connect with their inner child, offer healing, and provide love and support. This script can help address past trauma, emotional wounds, and provide comfort and nurturing from a present adult perspective.

Healing the Inner Child Hypnosis Script

Induction:

"Take a moment to get comfortable in your seat or lying down. Allow your body to relax deeply with each breath you take. Close your eyes, and begin to notice your breathing. Breathe in deeply, filling your lungs, and as you exhale, feel the tension begin to leave your body. Breathe in deeply again, and with each breath, you feel more and more relaxed, more at ease.

Let go of any thoughts or distractions. As you focus on your breathing, allow your body to become heavier and more relaxed. With each breath, allow yourself to drift deeper and deeper into a peaceful state of relaxation.

Now, I will count from 10 to 1. With each number, you will feel more and more relaxed, more and more at ease. 10... deeper and deeper relaxed... 9... releasing tension... 8... allowing your body to become calm and at peace... 7... feeling more and more comfortable... 6... you are safe and relaxed... 5... deeper still... 4... calm and peaceful... 3... feeling warm and relaxed... 2... completely at ease... 1... deeply relaxed, your mind calm and ready for healing."

Connecting with the Inner Child:

"Now that you are deeply relaxed, I want you to imagine that you are standing in front of a door. This door is special, and it leads to a room in your heart. On the other side of this door is a place where you can meet your inner child—the younger version of you who holds the memories and emotions of your early years.

This room is warm, welcoming, and safe. The door is open, and you are free to step inside at any time. When you are ready, take a step forward and walk into this peaceful space. As you do, you see yourself as a young child—perhaps you're standing at a particular age, or in a specific moment of your life that you feel called to visit. You are safe here, and there is no judgment.

Approach the child version of yourself and notice how they look. What is their age? What do they need? What is their expression? You may notice sadness, fear, or perhaps they are waiting for your love and attention. Allow yourself to move toward your inner child with compassion and love."

Healing and Nurturing the Inner Child:

"Now, as you stand in front of your inner child, I want you to understand that this child is an important part of who you are today. They carry the emotions, fears, joys, and experiences of your past, and they are seeking healing and comfort.

Imagine reaching out with kindness and tenderness to your inner child. Let them know that you are here now to offer them the love and care they may not have received in the past. You are here as the adult version of yourself, to nurture them, to provide what they need, and to reassure them that they are safe.

You can see the inner child looking up at you with trust and curiosity, knowing they are in good hands. Take a moment to hold them, comfort them, and let them know that they are loved. Speak gently and kindly to your inner child, offering words of healing and reassurance:

'You are safe. You are loved. You are not alone. I am here for you, and I will always protect you. You no longer have to carry the weight of the past. You are worthy of love, kindness, and peace. I'm here to take care of you now. It's time for you to feel safe and secure. You are free to let go of any pain, sadness, or fear. You can trust that I will always be here for you.'"

Releasing Old Wounds:

"Now, together with your inner child, take a moment to release any old wounds or fears that you may have been carrying. Imagine that any emotional pain or memories that are no longer serving you begin to dissolve and fade away. Picture the child letting go of sadness, fear, or any burdens they have been holding onto.

You might imagine the pain leaving as a dark cloud that slowly fades into the distance, or it might look like a weight being lifted from their shoulders. See this release, and feel the lightness and freedom that follows.

Now, with each exhale, you can feel these old emotions being released. Every breath you take brings healing and relief, and with each inhale, you are filling yourself with warmth, love, and acceptance."

Empowering the Inner Child:

"Now, I want you to focus on empowering your inner child. You are here now, as the adult you, and you can offer them all the strength, wisdom, and protection they need.

Imagine a bright, loving light filling your inner child's body. This light represents all the positive qualities you wish to nurture in them—self-love, confidence, courage, peace, and joy. Watch as this light fills them up, spreading warmth and comfort throughout their entire being.

Feel the child growing stronger and more confident as they accept these empowering qualities into their heart. You may even see them smiling, their posture becoming more confident and their energy becoming lighter and more at ease.

Now, speak to your inner child, offering words of encouragement:

'You are strong. You are worthy. You are enough, just as you are. You are capable of overcoming anything that comes your way. You have everything you need within you. I believe in you. You are precious, and you deserve all the love and happiness in the world.'"

Affirmations for Healing:

"Now, let's reinforce these feelings of love, strength, and healing with a few affirmations. As I say each affirmation, allow yourself and your inner child to repeat it, either silently or out loud:

- 'I love and accept myself unconditionally.'
- 'I forgive myself and release any pain from the past.'
- 'I am worthy of love, peace, and happiness.'
- 'I trust myself, and I trust my inner wisdom.'
- 'I am free to live a life of joy, love, and freedom.'
- 'I honor and cherish my inner child, and I offer them the love and support they need.'"

Integrating the Healing:

"Now that you've spent this time healing your inner child, take a moment to imagine bringing this energy of love, comfort, and healing back with you. You can carry this energy with you in your heart, and whenever you need, you can return to this place and offer your inner child love, support, and healing once again.

You and your inner child are now connected. You are not alone, and you will always have this support within you."

Awakening:

"In a moment, I will count from 1 to 5, and when I reach 5, you will return to full awareness, feeling calm, peaceful, and deeply healed.

1... slowly beginning to bring your awareness back to the present moment...

2... feeling refreshed and rejuvenated from the healing you have given your inner child...

3... bringing the energy of love, peace, and strength with you...

4... beginning to move your fingers and toes, gently waking your body...

5... fully awake, feeling peaceful, empowered, and ready to carry the love and healing of your inner child into the world with you."

This script guides the subject to connect with their inner child, nurture and heal emotional wounds, and provide loving, positive affirmation to support healing and growth. It's designed to help them move forward with a renewed sense of self-love and emotional well-being.

Next is a full *hypnosis script for connecting to a deceased loved one*, designed to facilitate a peaceful, healing experience where the person can feel connected to the memory and spirit of a loved one who has passed away. This script provides comfort, closure, and emotional healing while honoring the connection to the deceased.

Connecting to a Deceased Loved One Hypnosis Script

Induction:

"Begin by finding a comfortable position, either sitting or lying down. Allow your body to relax and your mind to become calm. Close your eyes, and take a deep breath in… and as you exhale, feel the tension begin to melt away. With each breath, you're becoming more and more relaxed, more at ease.

Let go of any thoughts, concerns, or distractions. Allow yourself to drift deeper and deeper with each breath. Imagine that each breath you take helps you relax even more, letting go of the stress and worries of the day. You're becoming more and more peaceful, more and more comfortable.

As you continue to breathe deeply, imagine a wave of relaxation sweeping over your body. It starts at the top of your head, and with each breath, this wave flows down your body, relaxing your scalp, your face, your neck, and shoulders. Let the relaxation flow down your arms, your chest, your abdomen, and your legs, all the way to your feet. You're feeling more and more relaxed, more at peace.

Now, I'm going to count from 10 to 1. With each number, you will feel yourself sinking deeper into relaxation, into a peaceful state of calm.

10… feeling more relaxed… 9… letting go of all tension… 8… your mind quieting… 7… deep relaxation… 6… feeling calm and at ease… 5… deepening even more… 4… completely relaxed and at peace… 3… deeper still… 2… almost at a perfect state of relaxation… 1… deeply relaxed, completely at ease."

Connecting to Your Deceased Loved One:

"Now, in this deeply relaxed state, you are ready to connect with the energy of your loved one. I want you to imagine that you are standing in a beautiful, peaceful place. It could be a place that feels familiar to you, or a place that feels completely new, but one that is calming and comforting. This is a place where time doesn't exist, and you are free to experience whatever you need.

In this special place, you see a gentle light in the distance. This light is warm, inviting, and peaceful. As you move closer to it, you begin to sense that it is connected to your loved one. It may feel like a glow, an aura, or a sense of presence that brings you comfort.

As you approach this light, you begin to sense your loved one's energy, a warmth that fills your heart with love and peace. And as you move closer, you notice that your loved one is standing there, waiting for you. You may see them clearly or feel their presence. You may even sense their energy without needing to see them fully. Know that whatever you are experiencing is just right for you. Allow yourself to feel the connection with them. You may feel their love, their presence, or even hear their voice. Take a moment to notice what you feel in this space."

Communication with Your Loved One:

"Now, in this sacred space, you have the opportunity to communicate with your loved one. They are here, and they are ready to listen and share with you. Take a moment to speak to them, either in your mind or aloud. You may wish to ask them any questions you have, express any feelings, or simply tell them what's in your heart.

Whatever you feel, know that this is a safe, loving, and healing space. Feel free to share your thoughts, memories, and emotions with them, knowing that they are listening with love and understanding.

(Allow some time for reflection or conversation here, depending on the depth of the session.)"

Receiving Messages or Healing:

"Now that you've shared your thoughts and feelings, take a moment to receive any messages, comfort, or healing that your loved one wishes to offer. They may speak to you directly, or you may receive messages in other forms—such as images, sensations, or emotions.

Trust the messages that come to you, knowing that your loved one is offering you guidance, reassurance, or simply love and peace. Feel free to accept this gift of love and healing from them."

(Allow the subject time to absorb the messages or healing offered by their loved one.)

Offering Healing and Closure:

"As you sit with your loved one, you may now feel the opportunity to offer them something in return—a message of love, forgiveness, or gratitude. Perhaps you want to say goodbye, or simply thank them for the impact they've had on your life.

Take this time to express your love, appreciation, and any final thoughts you wish to share. Know that these words are being received with love and that this moment is a beautiful, healing exchange."

Affirming the Connection:

"Even though you may leave this place today, know that the connection you share with your loved one is eternal. Their love, wisdom, and presence are always with you, and you can return to this space anytime you wish.

You may not always feel their physical presence, but know that their spirit is always with you, guiding you and offering you love and comfort whenever you need it."

Returning to the Present Moment:

"In a moment, I will count from 1 to 5. As I count, you will gradually begin to return to the present moment, bringing with you the love, healing, and peace from this experience.

1... slowly becoming aware of your surroundings...

2... taking a deep breath in, feeling refreshed and calm...

3... bringing back with you the love and healing from your loved one...

4... gently moving your fingers and toes, feeling awake and peaceful...

5... fully present, feeling grounded, and carrying the love of your loved one with you, always."

This script is designed to help the individual connect to their deceased loved one in a peaceful, healing way, offering comfort, closure, and the opportunity for emotional release. It's important that the subject is encouraged to trust the process, knowing that whatever they experience is valid and healing for them.

Next is complete *Forgiveness and Letting Go Hypnosis Script* designed to help a subject release emotional baggage, forgive others or themselves, and experience emotional freedom:

Forgiveness and Letting Go Hypnosis Script

Induction:

- Begin with a relaxation induction to guide the subject into a calm and focused state. Use a progressive relaxation method or any induction that you are comfortable with. Here is a simple example of a progressive relaxation induction:

_"Take a deep breath in... and as you breathe out, allow your body to relax... Just let go of any tension you might be carrying. Feel the muscles in your feet begin to relax... and with each breath, allow that relaxation to move slowly upwards. Let the relaxation flow into your ankles, your calves... feel the tension melting away from your knees, your thighs. Relax your hips, your lower back, and your stomach... Your chest becomes soft and at ease... Let the relaxation spread through your arms, your shoulders... down to your fingers, leaving them loose and relaxed. Let your neck and jaw relax, feel your face soften, your forehead smooth... Your whole body is relaxed, calm, and at peace.

Now, I want you to imagine a wave of relaxation gently sweeping down your back, all the way down to your feet, as if you're becoming completely relaxed and comfortable... with each breath, deeper and deeper into a peaceful, tranquil state. You are safe, comfortable, and completely at ease."_

Deepening the Trance:

- "With every breath you take, I'm going to count from 10 to 1... with each number, you'll feel yourself sinking deeper into a calm and peaceful state... 10... deeper and deeper... 9... allowing yourself to relax even further... 8... the relaxation flowing through every muscle, every nerve... 7... feeling more and more at ease... 6... the deeper you go, the better you feel... 5... completely relaxed... 4... deeper still... 3... almost there... 2... and 1... Now you're completely relaxed, deeply at peace, and open to this experience."_

Forgiveness and Letting Go Script:

- "Now that you are relaxed and comfortable, I want you to bring to mind someone with whom you may have experienced pain or hurt... this could be someone from your past or even yourself... it could be someone you're still holding anger or resentment toward... or even someone with whom you've never fully let go. Just allow yourself to bring this person to your awareness, but remember, you are in complete control. You can let go of any negative feelings at any time.

Imagine this person in front of you. As you see them, allow yourself to feel any emotion you've been holding onto, even if it's anger, sadness, or frustration... simply notice those emotions, but don't judge them. Just acknowledge them. You may notice that these emotions are connected to certain experiences or memories. Allow those memories to surface, but know that you are in control of how you respond.

Now, I want you to take a deep breath in... and as you breathe out, imagine all those negative emotions—anger, hurt, resentment—beginning to leave your body. With each exhale, the weight of those emotions is lightened.

See them float away, like leaves on a stream, moving further and further away from you. You no longer need to carry them. You have the power to release them."

- "Now, I want you to imagine a bright, healing light surrounding you. This light represents forgiveness. It is warm, gentle, and peaceful. It is a light that can heal wounds, release negative energy, and restore peace. See this light glowing all around you, filling your entire body with warmth and healing energy. Let it flow into your heart, your mind, and every part of your being.

As you sit in this light, I want you to imagine offering forgiveness... You don't need to justify or condone what was done. You simply need to release the power that these past events or actions have had over you. You are not forgiving the other person for them; you are forgiving for your own peace.

Take a moment and say in your mind, 'I forgive you for what you did. I release the hold this has had over me. I choose peace.' Notice how, with these words, the burden begins to lighten. Allow any remaining heaviness to melt away.

Now, repeat this process in your mind. 'I forgive myself. I release the guilt, the shame, and the pain. I choose to let go of these feelings and make space for love and healing.' With each breath, feel lighter, freer, and more at peace.

You are worthy of forgiveness, and you have the power to forgive, whether it's others or yourself. As you do this, notice the relief that comes, the peace that settles within you. You are free. You are no longer bound by the past. You are releasing it. And in this space of freedom, you are open to new possibilities of growth, love, and joy."

- "In this moment, you may also imagine the person or situation you are forgiving smiling at you, as if they too are grateful for this release. See them bathed in the same healing light, as if this energy of forgiveness also heals them.

Take a moment to simply feel the peace that comes with this release. Let it fill your heart.

With each breath, you grow more and more at peace, more and more aligned with the person you are meant to be—free, loving, and full of compassion. Now, with every breath, you feel even more free.

And as you do, know that forgiveness is a gift you give to yourself. You don't need to hold onto the past any longer. You are free, at peace, and ready to move forward in your life with love, understanding, and inner strength."

Reawakening:

- "Now, I'm going to begin counting from 1 to 5. As I do, you will gradually begin to come back to the present moment, feeling refreshed, calm, and at peace.

1... Slowly coming back... 2... bringing with you the feelings of peace and forgiveness... 3... noticing the room around you... 4... feeling energized and at ease... and 5... fully awake, feeling calm, refreshed, and light-hearted."

This script can be adapted and used for both individuals seeking to forgive others or themselves. The process of visualization, combined with relaxation and gentle suggestions, can lead to profound emotional releases. It's important that the subject is encouraged to take their time with these exercises and only proceed with forgiveness when they feel ready.

Finally, here is a *Motivation and Goal Achievement Hypnosis Script* designed to inspire action, clarity, and confidence in achieving personal goals:

Motivation and Goal Achievement Hypnosis Script

Induction:

- Start with a **progressive relaxation induction** to help the subject relax deeply.

_"Take a deep breath in... and slowly exhale... Allow your body to begin relaxing with each breath. Notice how the air feels as you breathe in... and how your body feels as you exhale, letting go of any tension.

Feel your feet and legs relaxing... Allow the tension to melt away from your hips, your stomach, your back... As you breathe deeply, your body becomes heavier, more relaxed with every breath.

Now, feel your shoulders, arms, and hands growing warm and relaxed... Let this feeling of peace and calm move up through your neck, your face... feel your whole body becoming soft and at ease. You are comfortable and relaxed.

With each breath, feel yourself sinking deeper and deeper into a state of deep relaxation... as if you are floating on a cloud, safe and calm. Your mind is open, receptive, and ready to make positive changes.

With every breath, you go deeper into a peaceful and relaxed state... more and more relaxed, deeper and deeper with each breath."_

Deepening the Trance:

- "Now, I will count down from 10 to 1... with each number, you will sink even deeper into relaxation... 10... going deeper still... 9... feeling more relaxed... 8... more at peace with each breath... 7... your mind and body are at ease... 6... drifting deeper... 5... halfway there... 4... completely relaxed... 3... deeply relaxed... 2... almost there... 1... now deeply relaxed, feeling calm, peaceful, and completely at ease."_

Motivation and Goal Achievement Script:

- "Now that you are deeply relaxed and focused, I want you to imagine yourself standing at the edge of a beautiful path. This path represents your journey to achieving your goals—your dreams. The way is clear, and ahead of you lies a future filled with success and accomplishment.

As you stand at the beginning of this path, take a moment to think about your most important goal—the one you want to achieve most. This is a goal that truly excites you, something that fills you with passion and purpose.

See this goal in your mind. Imagine what it looks like, how it feels. Visualize yourself already having achieved it, experiencing the joy and fulfillment that comes with success. Imagine the pride, the sense of accomplishment, the satisfaction you feel from reaching this goal. Allow yourself to feel these emotions fully. You've worked hard, and now you are experiencing the rewards.

Now, see yourself walking along this path toward your goal. With each step you take, feel yourself growing more confident, more motivated, and more focused. The closer you get, the clearer the path becomes, and the more you are filled with positive energy and determination.

As you walk this path, imagine any obstacles or challenges along the way. See them, but also see yourself easily overcoming them with strength, resourcefulness, and resilience. You have all the tools you need to succeed. You are capable, confident, and determined to move forward, no matter what.

Every challenge you encounter only makes you stronger and more focused on your goal. You know that nothing can stand in your way when you have the power of your will behind you.

With each breath, you are becoming more and more determined. You are filled with an unshakable belief in your ability to achieve your dreams. Your mind is clear, your heart is full of purpose, and your actions are aligned with your desires.

Now, I want you to imagine that you've reached your goal. See yourself standing at the finish line, feeling the excitement and sense of achievement. Know that you have already succeeded. It's yours. You've done it.

And with this feeling of success, you now feel even more motivated. You can see how the future is within your reach. You have the ability to create your desired outcome, and you are ready to take the necessary steps to get there.
Take a moment and really feel this success. Notice how it feels in your body, in your mind, and in your heart. This sense of accomplishment is yours to keep. It's real, and it's happening. With each passing day, you are getting closer to your goal."
Reinforcement of Motivation:

- "From now on, every day you wake up, you are filled with even more motivation to take the actions necessary to achieve your goals. You know that every small step forward is a step closer to success. You are confident, determined, and capable. Every decision you make brings you closer to the life you desire.

You are motivated by your passion, your vision, and your purpose. And with each day, your belief in yourself and your ability to succeed grows stronger.
You are already on the path to success. Each day, you take steps toward achieving your dreams, and every step brings you closer to the person you are meant to be. The more you focus on your goals, the more they become a reality. You will take the necessary actions, make the right choices, and find the strength within you to achieve everything you desire."
Awakening:

- "In a moment, I will count from 1 to 5. As I count, you will begin to return to the present moment, bringing with you the motivation, confidence, and clarity you've experienced today. You will feel refreshed, alert, and ready to take on the world, filled with energy and enthusiasm for your goals.

1... beginning to return... 2... feeling the energy returning to your body... 3... you're becoming more aware of your surroundings... 4... starting to feel awake and alert... and 5... fully awake, feeling motivated, confident, and ready to take action toward your goals."

This *Motivation and Goal Achievement script* can be customized to target specific goals (e.g., career success, personal growth, fitness) and can also be used for recurring motivation or boosting self-confidence. It aims to instill a sense of purpose, self-belief, and momentum, helping the subject feel empowered and ready to take practical steps toward their aspirations.

Epilogue: The Journey Beyond

As you close the final pages of this book, remember that this is not the end of your journey with hypnosis—it is only the beginning. The knowledge and techniques you've gained are powerful tools that will continue to evolve as you put them into practice. Every session, every person you work with, and every moment you dedicate to mastering the art of hypnosis will deepen your understanding of the limitless potential within the human mind.

Hypnosis is not merely a set of techniques; it is a profound connection between the conscious and the subconscious, a bridge that enables true transformation. In mastering hypnosis, you are not just learning how to guide others—you are unlocking the potential within yourself. The deeper you go into this craft, the more you will uncover about your own mind, your own limitations, and your ability to create lasting change.

For those of you stepping into hypnosis as a professional, know that you are entering a field where the most profound, lasting change happens at the level of the subconscious. Your role as a practitioner is one of profound responsibility. You are not just offering suggestions; you are facilitating healing, empowering individuals to break free from patterns that no longer serve them, and helping them embrace their fullest potential. The work you do will ripple outward, affecting not only the individuals you work with but their families, their communities, and beyond. Each breakthrough, each transformation, will become a testament to the power of the mind to heal, grow, and evolve.

For those of you seeking personal transformation through hypnosis, know that you hold within you the ability to access deep reserves of wisdom, strength, and creativity. The tools you now have at your disposal—whether for stress relief, habit change, or personal empowerment—are just the start. By continuing to work with the subconscious mind, you will uncover new depths of possibility and resilience, discovering a version of yourself that is free from limiting beliefs and open to all the opportunities life has to offer.

The mind is a vast, untapped frontier. As you move forward with your practice, always remember that the journey is not about reaching a destination, but about embracing the process of discovery. Hypnosis invites you to explore the unseen, to question what you thought you knew about yourself and the world around you, and to open the door to a more vibrant, empowered life.

And so, the work you've begun here will continue to unfold. Whether you are using hypnosis for personal growth, helping others heal, or delving into new areas of study, know that this path is one of endless potential. The tools you now have at your fingertips—combined with your dedication, your curiosity, and your openness to growth—will allow you to step into a future where anything is possible.

Continue to explore, continue to practice, and continue to unlock the power of the mind. This is just the beginning of a remarkable journey—one that will change not only the lives of those you touch but also your own life in ways you have yet to imagine.

Thank you for taking the first step toward mastering hypnosis. The mind is waiting for you to unlock its full potential. Go forth and change the world—one mind at a time.

About Alex Telman

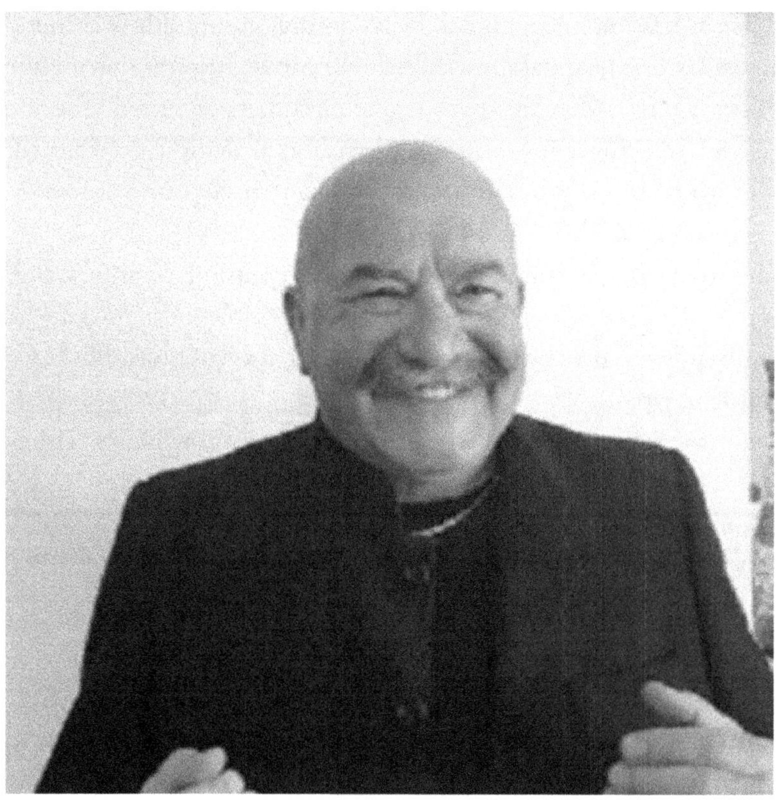

Alex Telman is a globally recognized spiritual healer, author, and one of the country's most read poets. With over 45 years of experience, he has dedicated his life to helping individuals break free from negative energies, trauma, and spiritual blockages. His transformative work has empowered a diverse range of clients, including celebrities, business leaders, educators, and everyday individuals, guiding them toward emotional well-being, personal growth, and spiritual fulfillment.

From an early age, Alex demonstrated extraordinary abilities to perceive and remove harmful energies and entities, a gift that first emerged when he was just three years old. This rare talent led him to study with psychic masters across the globe—Afghanistan, France, Sweden, Israel, England, and Australia—each recognizing his unique gifts and helping him refine his craft.

In addition to his healing practice, Alex has practiced as a barrister, teacher, university lecturer, and small business owner, offering a well-rounded perspective on healing that combines spirituality with practical action. He is also an accomplished author, whose writings inspire and uplift readers by exploring the depths of human emotion and the power of self-healing.

Through his sessions, Alex has helped countless individuals overcome emotional turmoil and reclaim their lives. His work transcends cultural and geographical boundaries, offering profound healing to those in need. His mission is simple yet powerful: to guide people back to their authentic selves, helping them live with purpose, peace, and fulfillment.

With a career built on compassion, wisdom, and deep spiritual insight, Alex remains a beacon of hope for anyone seeking to overcome their struggles and wanting to step into a life of clarity and joy.

Other Titles by Alex Telman

Non Fiction

From Cursed to Cured: 100 True Stories of Healing from Curses
Connecting to the Afterlife: a how-to guide
Your Journey from Death to Rebirth
Empower Your Sundays: Unlocking Inner Strength for a Resilient Life
The Truth Behind the Creation Story: A Journey Through Reincarnation
Practical Mentalism in a Nutshell
Reprogram Your Mind in a Nutshell
Meditation in a Nutshell
Alex Telman in Quotes

Novels

Down and Out in Byron Bay
One Life, Half Lived
Homeless in New York
God Speaks: A Journey Through Creation in His Own Words
Jesus Speaks: The Man Behind the Miracle in His own Words

Poetry

Echoes of September 11
Burning Echoes of Time
From Dawn to Dusk: the life cycle in sonnets
Eternal Echoes: The Tapestry of Time and the Unseen
Snapshots of People I Have Never Met
Legends and Lessons: 36 Myths Unveiled
A Measure of Time: The Eternal Voyage of Self

Ashes of Verses: Poems Burned But Not Forgotten
Telman: The Complete Haiku 1974-2024
Reflections on Solitude: A Poetic Journey Through The Lonely Mind
Your Friendship is a Museum
Whispers to Bella

Don't miss out!

Visit the website below and you can sign up to receive emails whenever Alex Telman publishes a new book. There's no charge and no obligation.

https://books2read.com/r/B-A-YBSCC-XUEKF

Connecting independent readers to independent writers.